SOLO CAMINO

SOLO CAMINO

An Empowering Guide for Women

Renée Hartleib

HeartWrite Press

Solo Camino: An Empowering Guide For Women
Copyright © 2025 Renée Hartleib

First published in 2025
HeartWrite Press

ISBN 978-1-7781979-2-5

Requests for information should be addressed to:
renee@reneehartleib.com

All rights reserved. No part of this book may be used or reproduced in any manner without prior written permission except in the case of brief quotations embodied in reviews.

Cover and interior design by Megan Sheer
sheerbookdesign.com

*Malve, for all the ways you helped me get there,
and for all the ways you return me home,
this book is for you.*

CONTENTS

Introduction	1
Preface	7
Part 1: What is Standing in Your Way?	**11**
Safety	13
Confidence	17
Societal Conditioning	19
Inner Critic	21
Age	25
Fitness	27
Money	29
Time	31
Are You Ready For Your Wander?	33
Part 2: Choose Your Path and Pack Your Bag	**37**
Discover Your Why	39
Set Your Own Intentions	41
Make Your Big Decisions	45
Book Your Planes and Trains	49
Get Your Body Ready	51
Plan and Research	55
Learn the Language	59
Pack Your Bag	61
Prepare Your Feet	65
Pick Your Poles	69
Investigate Technology	71
Keep a Journal	75

Part 3: The Journey Itself: What I Learned on My Camino   77

  The Beginning   79
    Stepping Out   81
    Expecting the Unexpected   85
    Listening to Your Body   89
    Respecting Your Own Nature   93
    Honouring Connections   95
    Feeding Yourself   99
    Going Off-Stage   103
    Keeping Your Eyes Up   107
    Taking Care of Business   109

  The Middle   113
    Finding Humour   115
    Enjoying the Mornings   117
    Choosing Water Over Wine   119
    Reaching for Joy   123
    Allowing Rest Days   127
    Coping With Heat   129
    Overcoming Challenges   133
    Battling the Inner Critic   137
    Avoiding Bedbugs   141
    Embracing Perspective   143

  Nearing the End   145
    Letting Go   147
    Walking in the Rain   149
    Staying Open   151
    Speaking Your Truth   153
    Going with the Flow   157
    Dealing with Disillusionment   159

Giving and Receiving News	161
Encountering Camino Angels	163
Finishing Your Solo Camino	167

Part 4: The Path Continues: After Your Camino — 171

Including Buffer Time	173
Seeking Meaning	175
Dealing with Contradictory Emotions	177
Accepting Your Unique Camino	179
Practising Patience	183
Sharing Your Camino	185
Celebrating Yourself	189
Planning the Next One!	191
In Closing	193
Spread the Word	195
Gratitude	197
Resources	199

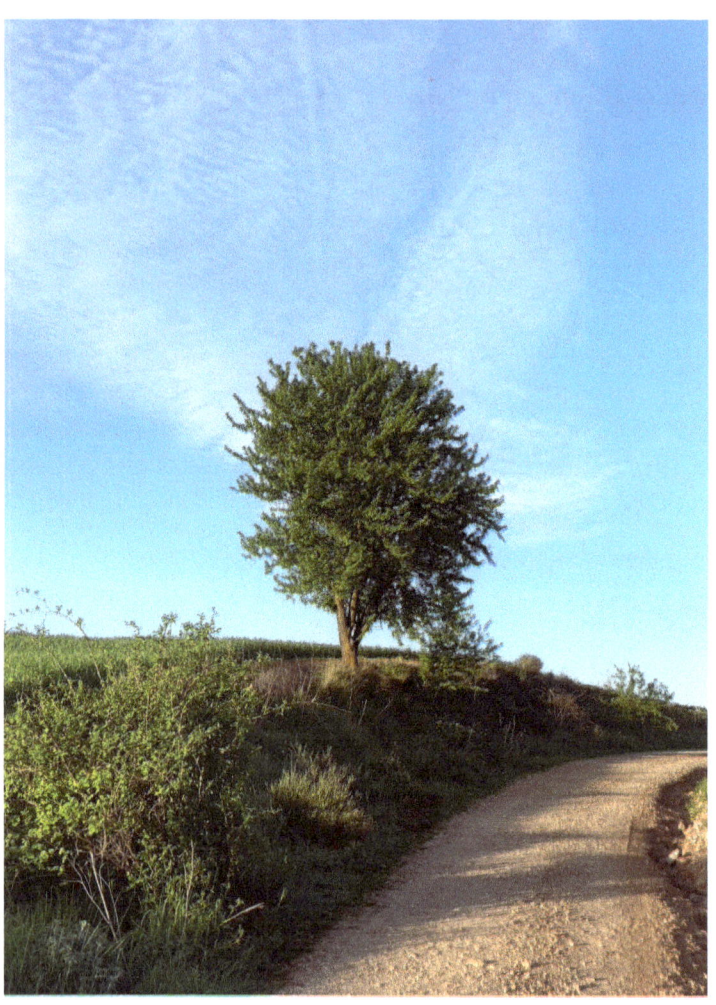

INTRODUCTION

If you're a woman dreaming of completing a long walk, such as the Camino de Santiago in Spain, and doing it alone, this book is for you! It is meant to inspire you and empower you to organize and undertake this type of adventure on your own.

When I first started dreaming about walking the Camino, I knew it was important to go on my own. Having never taken a solo trip, I longed for an opportunity to do something big that was just for me. I didn't want to have to factor another person into my decisions. It would be a trip that was for me and about me—sometimes a novel concept for women!

Does this resonate with you? We all have different reasons for wanting to go solo. You might be someone who has spent years taking care of aging parents and children or who everyone turns to for help and guidance. Maybe you're an introvert who doesn't get enough time alone. Or perhaps you're someone who has had her share of "unwanted journeys"—divorce, death, illness—and who yearns for time alone to make sense of all that has happened.

Whatever your situation and whatever your reason for wanting to set out on a solo trip, my hope is that this book will give you necessary information plus some good first-person stories that will help build your confidence. And if you have always wanted to do it but have had "cold feet," it will also encourage you to examine what might be holding you back.

Solo Camino: An Empowering Guide for Women came out of my walk on the Camino Francés in Spain in the spring of 2024. It had long been a dream that I was finally able to realize. And when I arrived and began walking, to my surprise, there was one question that I fielded repeatedly.

"You're doing this alone?" It was always asked by women and often with an air of incredulity, followed up quickly by a series of statements that sounded something like this:

"I could never do this alone."

"Aren't you afraid?"

"I wanted to do it alone but didn't think I could, so I waited for my best friend/sister/partner/husband to do it with me."

Does any of this sound familiar? Do safety concerns, as a woman alone, stop you? Maybe you lack confidence in yourself? Or is it the fear of the unknown that gives you pause? If the answer is yes to any of these questions, read on!

THE BOOK IS SPLIT INTO FOUR PARTS:

PART ONE explores your desire to go on a walking adventure and the practical or emotional hurdles that might stand in the way of moving forward with that dream.

PART TWO is all about preparing for your long walk with loads of practical advice. When will you go? How many kilometres will you cover? What will you pack?

PART THREE covers the journey itself and what you can expect. It includes my own personal Camino stories and tips on accommodation, language, heat, rain, and gear. I'll also talk about ways to take care of your body and spirit.

PART FOUR readies you for returning home and gives you some insight on what might happen after a trip like this, complete with self-care advice.

Throughout the book, I offer you questions to mull over as you plan your journey. If you are inclined to put pen to paper, you can use them as writing prompts. Sometimes an additional layer of clarity emerges when we write, rather than simply thinking about a question. I've included these prompts for reflection where I believe they would be most useful to you.

This is the kind of book I wish I'd had when I was preparing for my Camino—something written specifically for women, with all the information in one place. A book that doesn't just give a glossy "It's so great" narrative, but one that actually talks in real terms about some of the challenges you may face, both emotionally and physically.

While many of the concepts about solo travel in this book can be applied on any journey you do alone, all of my specific examples are related to the Camino (because this is the route I walked). If you are keen to set out on another path, I would advise that you search for specific resources related to the long-distance walk, pilgrimage, or adventure you have in mind.

You *can* do this on your own. I'm here to tell you it's possible! And be prepared for a big payoff. I truly believe, and have learned from my own experience, that when we clear space in our lives just for us, and when we respect ourselves enough to put our own needs first, much personal growth follows.

When you decide to pursue a solo Camino or another adventure, you have so much to look forward to: not only a beautiful connection with yourself, but also a huge sense of pride, accomplishment, and vigour that comes at the end of fulfilling a dream and doing it on your own terms.

Let's dive in!

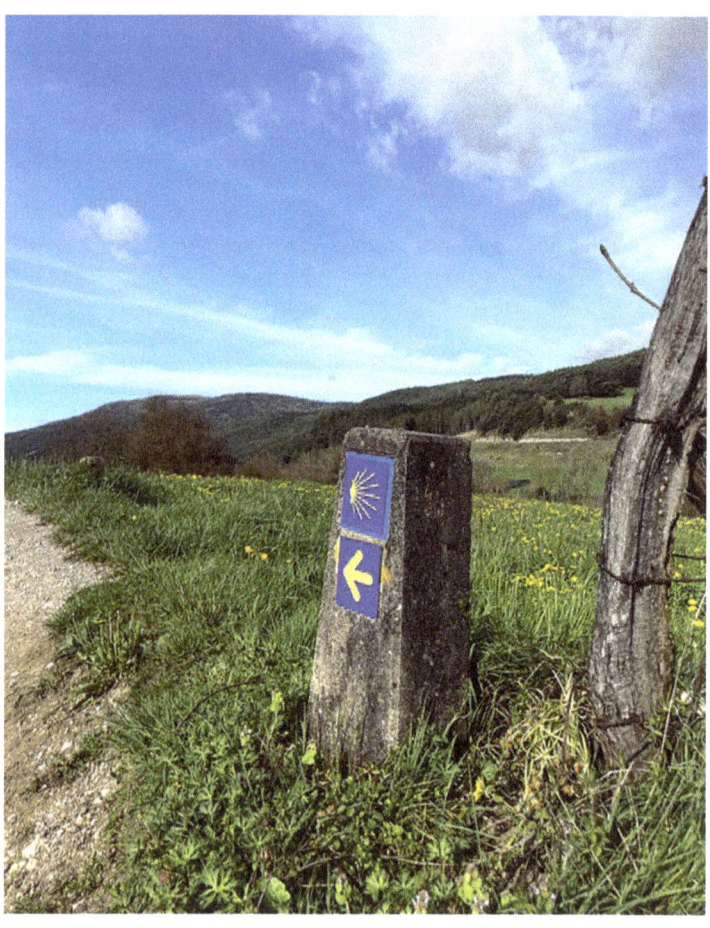

INTRODUCTION

THIS BOOK IS FOR YOU IF:

You are a woman longing for a solo walking adventure, whether it's for spiritual, physical, or emotional reasons.

You are interested in walking the Camino Francés, a different Camino route in Europe, or a long-distance walk in another part of the world.

You are being held back from a solo adventure by fear or uncertainty.

You would like to have the confidence to embark on a journey on your own and don't want to wait for a family member or friend to go with you.

You dream of relying on your own smarts, will, and competency to make your vision of a big trip a reality.

You want to hear stories about another woman's solo experience.

You want more information about preparing for and executing long walking journeys.

You have already done a Camino and want to reflect on your experience and perhaps plan another walk!

WHAT THIS BOOK ISN'T:

A guidebook. There are so many guidebooks to choose from, with maps, information about topography and distance, plus climate and local customs. I would highly recommend you buy one of these for your chosen route. They are usually quite small and light and are something you can take with you and consult as you walk your way.

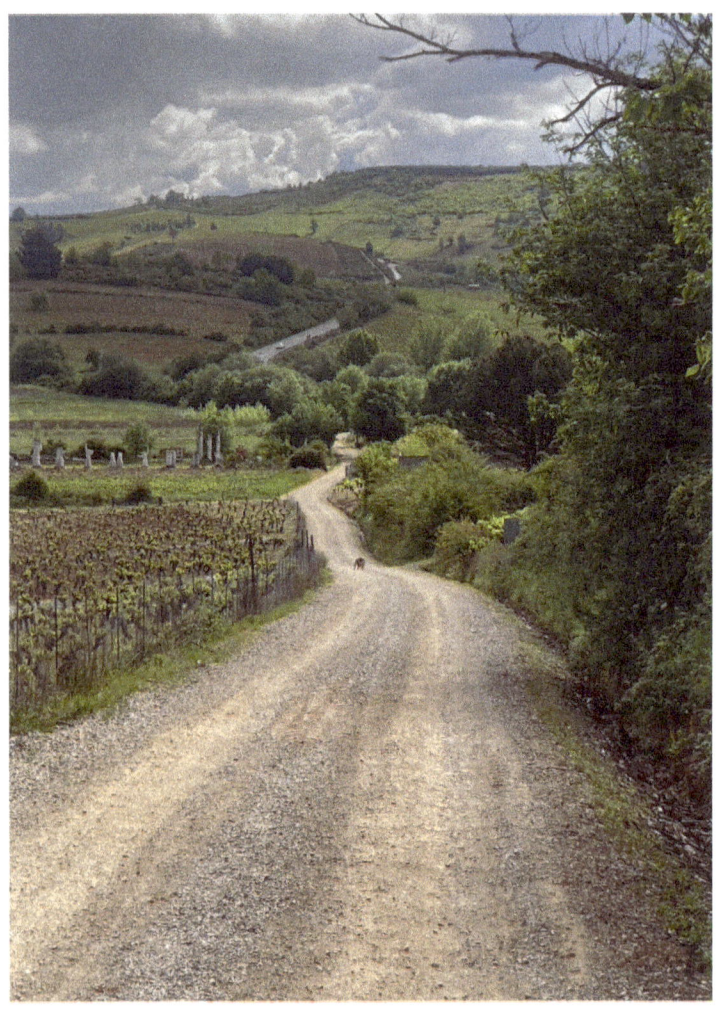

PREFACE

It might start with a book or a movie or a song, or with a story overheard. It may feel like a small tug on your heart, a pull you feel in your body, or a call that you need to answer. I'm talking about the impulse to walk the Camino de Santiago in Spain, or another pilgrimage path or long-distance walk anywhere in the world.

What is this mysterious draw? Where does it come from? And why can't so many of us shake it?

My first exposure to the Camino was through Shirley MacLaine's book *The Camino*, way back in the '80s. I had never heard of the path she walked before I read the book, and I was intrigued. A long walk—across almost a whole country—that had a spiritual element and that scores of other people had done throughout history. An ancient pilgrimage trail that has religious roots, and some say pagan ones as well.

Fast forward to 2009, and I was alone in a car listening to CBC, Canada's national broadcaster. I had tuned in halfway through an instrumental piece of music that had the sound of footsteps and cow bells and church bells, on top of soulful violin. I found myself moved by the music and crying without being able to understand why, but I knew enough to write down the name of the composer when the song ended.

Oliver Schroer. And the album was called *Camino*. I learned that the tunes on the album were recorded in churches along the way when he walked the Camino in 2004. I also learned that Schroer had died of leukemia at age fifty-two, only four years after he completed his journey. I bought the CD (people still did that then!), and when I listened to it, it seemed to pluck a secret string inside me, one that I didn't know the length or shape or colour of.

And then *The Way*, the movie with Martin Sheen, directed by his son Emilio Estevez, came out the following year, and I cried my eyes out the first time I watched it. And the second time as well. Ah, there it is again, I thought. This strangely emotional pull to the idea of walking the Camino.

But at the time, I had a small child and was recently separated, so the Camino seemed like a dream for another time. I told myself I would go when I turned fifty, but that time came and went too; I had recently entered a new relationship and had also quit drinking, both of which were fresh starts that required energy.

And then one day, in 2021, my partner, Malve, and I were out on a long hike and I was talking about doing the Camino, the way I did from time to time. She turned to me and said: "You know, if you really want to do a big trip like that, you need to set a date." She was right, of course. You can't keep saying you want to do something but never set aside the time. In that moment, I decided to do the Camino in 2024, the year after my daughter was set to graduate from high school.

I spoke it out loud, and my planning began.

I tell you this story to connect with you and to help you feel not so alone. If you've picked up my book, you probably feel a similar urge for a grand solo adventure, and maybe, like me, you have put it off or dismissed it in some way.

PREFACE

In what ways do you feel called? And is it time for you to answer your own call?

Hearing Oliver Schroer's music and feeling such emotion, without knowing the album was related to the Camino, still feels wonderful and mysterious to me. This memory, and everything that has happened since then, makes me believe there is a larger, invisible force at work, one that nudges us in certain directions. Something inside of us that says YES. And it's up to us to pay attention, to listen, and to respond.

In the pages ahead, we'll acknowledge this urge you are feeling for your own solo Camino and explore what might be holding you back. Because when we know we're being called but we don't do anything about it, there's likely something standing in the way.

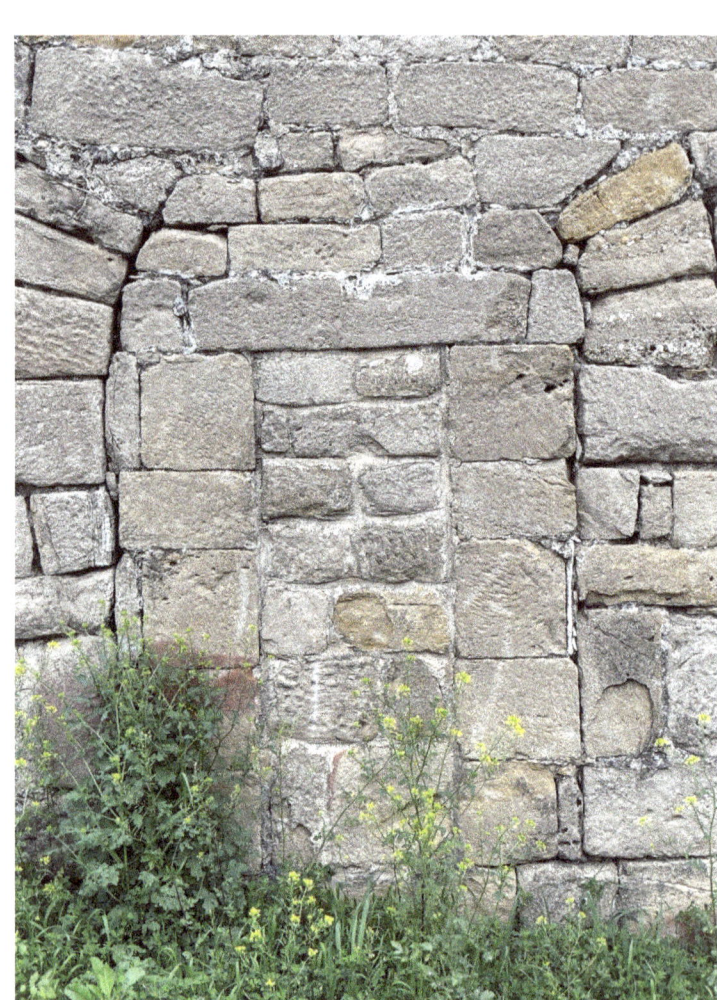

PART ONE

WHAT IS STANDING IN YOUR WAY?

If you picked up this book called *Solo Camino*, there is a part of you that very much wants to make this journey on your own. I understand that. It's what I wanted too. But if you haven't yet started stepping toward your goal, what is holding you back?

For many women, the big stopper is the question of safety. But if you follow that fear a little deeper, you may find something more nuanced: a lack of confidence, perhaps, or a belief that a solo trip is selfish.

As women, we often spend our lives taking care of other people. For some of us, this "caretaker" persona feels like our identity. Therefore, a big expenditure of time, energy, and cash might feel extravagant or excessive on a trip that is just for ourselves.

Other roadblocks may be our fitness level, our age, how much money we have at our disposal, or not enough vacation time. I've talked to a lot of women who, although drawn to a trip like the Camino, say things like:

"I think I missed my opportunity—I'm too old now," or "I just can't take that kind of time away from my family or my work," or "I can barely walk around the block without huffing or puffing—how would I walk all the way across Spain?"

In the short chapters ahead, we'll tackle the most common fears, worries, and blocks that may be stopping you from striding toward your goal.

REFLECTION / WRITING PROMPTS:

How has the Camino, or another walking adventure, called to you? When was the first time you heard about it? How persistent has the nudge to take this trip been?

What has stopped you from doing it so far? What has been holding you back? Be specific.

SAFETY

I think safety is likely Fear #1 when it comes to women and solo adventures. And no wonder. We've been taught, since we were just small girls, that there are all kinds of places women should never be alone—from dark alleys to deserted parking lots to foreign countries. We've also been instructed that having a man, or another person, with us at all times keeps us safer.

To counter this narrative, here are some reassuring facts about the Camino routes in Spain:

The Camino is one of the safest places you could travel and walk as a woman.

This is my opinion, so please do your own research. Consider looking into the safety stats on the Camino and compare them with the place you live or other places you have travelled or might travel as a woman alone. You will probably be surprised. Having walked the Camino myself, I can honestly say that as a woman, I felt safer than I do in most big cities, or in other parts of the world where I've travelled. Also, if seeing police officers or police cars brings you reassurance, I noticed a subtle but consistent police presence, even in rural areas.

Depending on what time of year you take your trip, you will likely rarely be fully alone.

If you choose to walk the Camino Francés, there are villages every few kilometres, and except during the winter months of November–February, it is well populated with walkers. There may be some sections of the path where you are completely alone, but more often than not, you will see someone in front of you or behind you at all times. In addition, there is a solid infrastructure of lodging, restaurants, and other public places, so you definitely won't be wandering around trying to find food or someplace to sleep as night is falling. Some of the other Camino routes have less developed infrastructure and fewer pilgrims, so you will need to assess your own comfort level with what is available.

There is an air of goodwill along the Camino.
Strangers checking in on you when you stop to rest. Someone cheering you on from the sidelines when you're struggling. Locals pointing you in the right direction. These are just some of the simple but thoughtful acts of kindness you will encounter on the Camino. Knowing that the locals and the other people on the path truly have your back leads to a beautiful sense of community and safety.

Every year, more and more women are walking.
Since 2017, the number of women walking the Camino has increased dramatically. In fact, the latest statistics show that 53 percent of the pilgrims who make it to Santiago are women. While on the path, I met many other women who were doing the journey solo, each with her own unique reasons.

All of this is not to say that there aren't risks to women walking alone on the Camino, or anywhere in the world. There is always the risk of sexual harassment or sexual assault. We must weigh the

SAFETY

risks and take necessary precautions, but I believe we should not allow this fear to stop us cold.

Some of these precautions could be taking a self-defence course, investing in an eSIM card with unlimited data for your phone (more on this in Part Two), and acquainting yourself with what to do—and what number to call—in case of an emergency. In addition, consider joining an online forum or a Camino group specifically for women; if they hear of a danger to women, they publish timely warnings about areas to avoid.

If the Camino isn't your jam and you're looking to do another type of walk or adventure elsewhere in the world, do your research! Rather than letting fear stop you from doing something you really want to do, consider what would help make you feel safer instead.

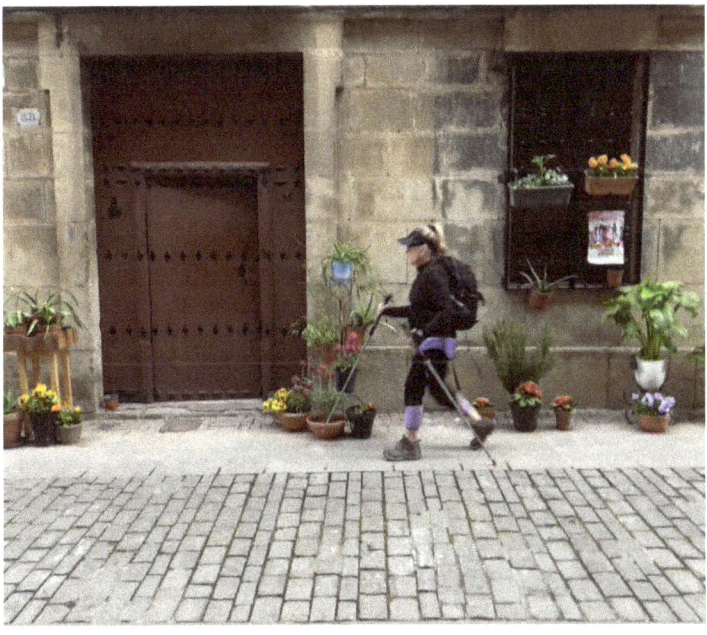

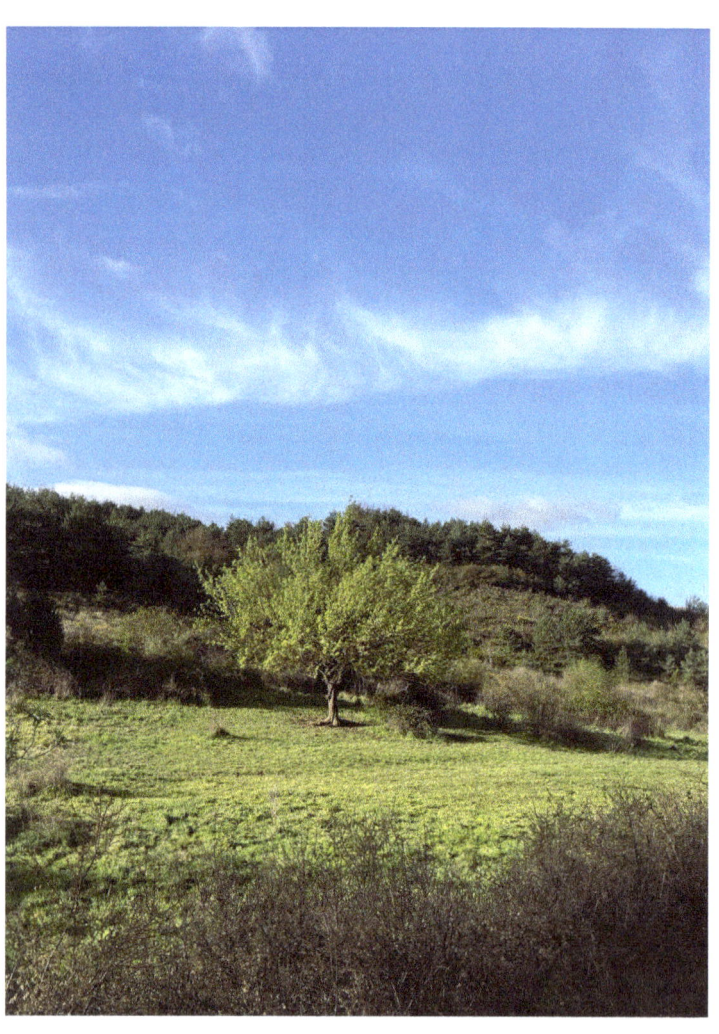

CONFIDENCE

None of us are perfectly confident in every area of life. You might feel super confident when it comes to balancing your financial books, but you don't like walking into a room full of strangers. You may find it easy to change the tires on your car but feel nervous about making Christmas dinner. Or you might be able to plan all of your kid's play dates and negotiate home care for your elders but lack confidence when it comes to planning a trip of your own.

In addition, if you're in a relationship with another person and you are used to doing things together, it might seem like a big leap to undertake this kind of a trip by yourself. There are a lot of puzzle pieces that need to fit together—transportation, research, training, preparation—and this can feel intimidating if you've never done something like this on your own before.

If you recognize that a lack of confidence is standing in your way, get curious. And get specific. What part are you most nervous about, and what you can do to soothe this anxiety? Are there practical steps you can take? Is there support you can receive? For instance, if you feel nervous about becoming ill while travelling, just checking out the details of health or travel insurance might make you feel more secure.

Remember, confidence is a learned skill. We aren't born with it. We can grow our confidence in any area we choose, including solo trips to wonderful places where we challenge our bodies and provide joy to our spirits!

REFLECTION / WRITING PROMPTS:

Be specific about your lack of confidence when it comes to planning this kind of a big trip. What parts feel scary or overwhelming?

Is there anything practical you can do to increase your confidence in these areas?

What can you do to soothe yourself? Is there someone else who can support you?

SOCIETAL CONDITIONING

Most of us have lives where, in addition to working full-time, we also look after families and homes and elders and pets. The Camino offers a chance to shut the door on all of that and simply look after ourselves and the few items we are carrying with us.

But you need to leave home before you can start enjoying this freedom. And that's where many women get stopped. Putting yourself first, in the form of a big trip like this, might make you uncomfortable. It might also feel like too big of an ask for those who depend on you.

Let's push back on this a little and add some context.

As women, we have been conditioned by our societal systems to provide for others and play a caretaking role. That's why, when we consider planning a big solo trip just for ourselves, discomfort and a fear of selfishness may naturally arise.

We may have also been taught to place ourselves second, behind all those other people we're looking after. Maybe you're a kick-ass doer and an absolute superstar at taking care of everyone else, but your own needs and self-care come last. You might even convince yourself that you're indispensable and worry if you ever went away for a significant period of time, your family would starve or fall apart without you.

If you play a specific caretaking role within your family, workplace, or broader community, you may need to challenge yourself to adopt a different perspective and give yourself permission to fulfill a dream that takes you away for a chunk of time.

Food for thought: You deserve the same type of love and care you so freely give to others. You are allowed to do something that is just for you. You are worthy of a trip that grants you the space and time to be yourself and to take care of yourself.

REFLECTION / WRITING PROMPTS:

Based on societal conditioning and the role you play in your family, do you feel you are being held back from a journey like the Camino? Explain how.

Do you also sense that you are holding yourself back from taking this big step? If so, how does that manifest?

What kind of tools are at your disposal to challenge societal conditioning and broaden your own sense of possibility? Can these tools assist you and be carried with you on your Camino?'

INNER CRITIC

The negative and critical voice in our heads can sometimes be our worst enemy, especially when it comes to dreams or ideas that will change our norm or "rock the boat."

Having an intense inner critic myself, I have spent years trying to understand this aspect of our human selves. In fact, I devoted an entire chapter to the topic in my first book, *Writing Your Way: A 40-Day Path of Self Discovery*. Here's part of what I wrote:

> First things first: We all have an inner critical voice. No one is immune or exempt. But we all have our own unique version of this voice that is connected to how we were raised.
>
> Psychologists say that our inner critic forms in childhood as we ingest parental and societal messages about how to be in the world. When we are cautioned about behaviours that might cause us to be ostracized or rejected, we internalize that information and create a belief system of our own. Basically, the role of the inner critic is to spare us shame by warning us when we begin to enter potentially "dangerous territory."
>
> It's ironic that something that developed to help us avoid the negative emotion of shame actually causes shame. Our inner critic shouts, calls us names, and is often down-

right vicious. This part of us is also sneaky, crafting critical words to sound like the truth. The truth that other people are too polite to say; that's what we tell ourselves.

Our inner critic likes to give opinions about almost everything: how we look, the work we do, the work we don't do, what we just said, what we didn't say, and what kind of parents and partners and people we are. Our critic is convinced we're not smart enough, attractive enough, cool enough, creative enough, or organized enough. In fact, according to our critic, we're just not "enough," period!

Attempting a long-distance walk in a foreign country *by yourself* certainly falls into the category of boat-rocking and dangerous territory. I'd be surprised if your inner critic hasn't made an appearance yet!

When you consider doing the Camino, is there a voice from inside you that is keen to shoot the whole idea down? Does it even sound a little bit mean?

A very important thing to remember is that your inner critic is NOT the voice of the truth. It's an ancient part of us that is actually trying to protect us, even if its specific ideas about how to do so are misguided. But, we have agency and we are allowed to redirect it.

Therefore, *You're out of shape, you'll make a fool of yourself* could be countered with *People with all different body types and from all walks of life do the Camino. I will fit right in and get stronger as I go*!

You're not organized enough to do this on your own can be transformed into *I trust that I am able to take good care of myself.*

And *You're not strong enough to walk that far, and what if something happens?* can become *If I find myself in a situation that is unsafe or where I'm hurt, I know that I can take care of it. And I also know how to ask for help.*

INNER CRITIC

REFLECTION / WRITING PROMPTS:

What do you tell yourself about your ability to do this long walk? Is your inner voice serving you when you think about the Camino, or is it holding you back?

If it's currently holding you back, how might you change the dialogue in your head to something more helpful?

Practise countering old, outdated, or inaccurate beliefs with a kinder and more compassionate message that gives you room to try something new and succeed!

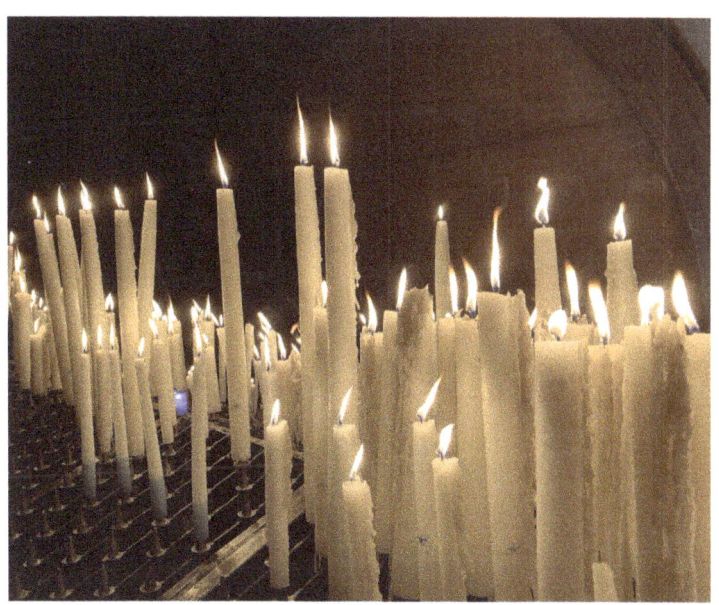

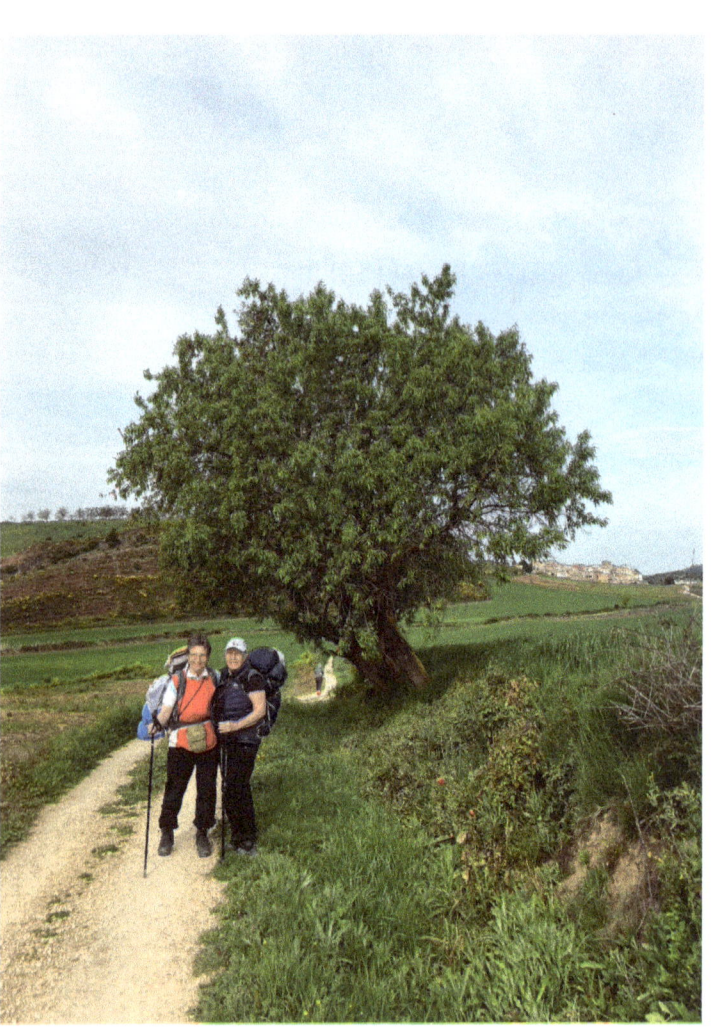

AGE

The Camino is not just a young person's game. Not at all! It's definitely an all-ages venue with a beautiful mix of people from teens to young families to mid-lifers to retirees. When I walked, I really took notice of the great number of mature walkers, those in their late sixties, seventies, and even eighties. And a lot of them seemed in better shape than I was!

Our ideas of what we might be capable of often come from our parents and what we witnessed them doing at certain ages. How physically fit were your parents when they were the age you are now? I feel lucky that I saw my mom power walking when she was in her fifties. At the time, she could walk much faster than I could, and I was barely thirty!

What I most want to say about age is not to let the idea of a number, or what you may have (falsely) learned about the constraints of age, hold you back. If you really want to take yourself on this adventure, assess your fitness level, talk with your doctor or naturopath about anything you might be worried about, and look into what it would take for you to prepare to fulfill your dream.

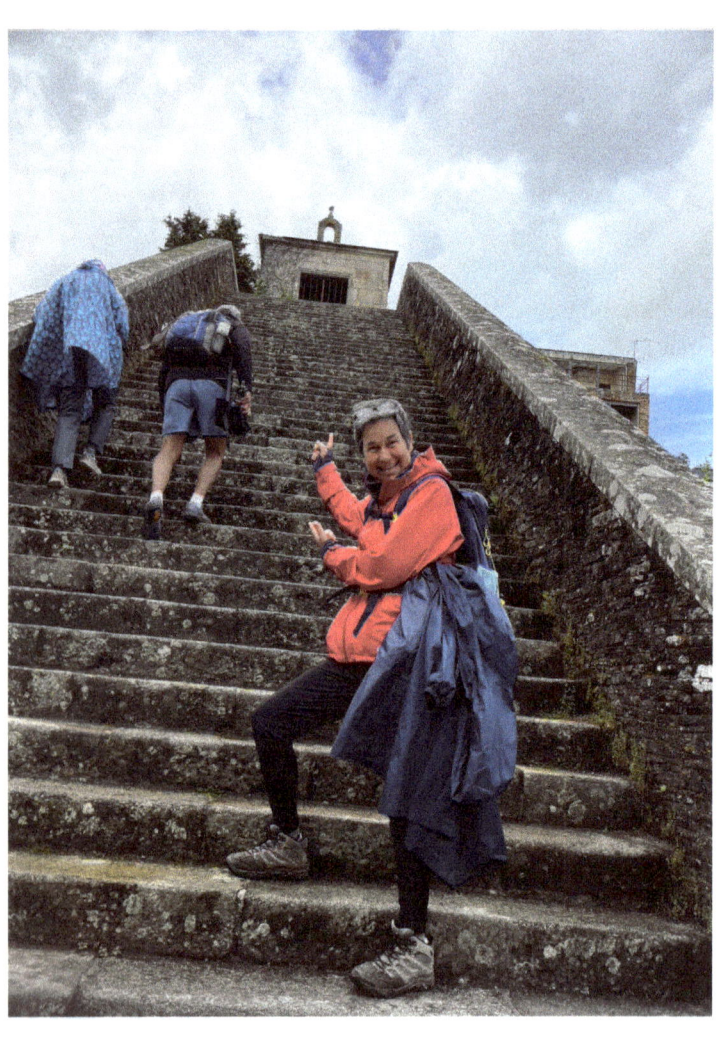

FITNESS

If you can walk, you can do the Camino—because walking is all it is. *But wait a minute*, you might say, *don't I need to walk long distances? Aren't there lots of hills?*

Yes, there are hills and yes, you'll need to walk some long distances, but you can work on your fitness level prior to embarking on your trip. If this is something you really want to make happen, there is much you can do to physically ready yourself (more on this in Part Two). And all of that preparation will help you feel more confident about the journey. Consider getting some professional advice from a physiotherapist or an osteopath prior to your walk. I did this and ended up investing in a pair of orthotics that were a godsend both for my training and the actual walk itself.

You can also pace yourself on the Camino. If you have more time at your disposal, you don't have to do a lot of long-distance days back to back. Shorter days and more rest days, especially at the beginning, can really help if you're worried about your fitness level. If you have more time and want to take it really slow, I would encourage you to do that.

Lastly, don't make the mistake of thinking that a persistent injury or joint pain is a stopper. I met lots of people who had "areas of weakness," and they took care of themselves, only doing what they could. For instance, a number of people I met who had pre-existing knee trouble used a luggage transfer service for their backpacks. They knew their knees couldn't take the extra weight, so they paid four or five Euros a day to have their bag picked up and delivered.

Same goes for chronic health conditions—it doesn't mean a trip like this is off-limits. You can work with your health care provider to ensure you have enough medication for the whole trip. (Don't forget to create a list of medications or prescriptions you can present to a pharmacist just in case what you've brought along gets lost!)

Before you make your current fitness level or any pre-existing conditions a stopper, learn how your body responds to longer-form walking, and figure out how you can best support yourself.

MONEY

The great thing about the Camino is that if money is an issue, you can actually do it very inexpensively. Your biggest outlay of cash, depending on where you live, will be the transportation to get there, plus some fundamental Camino supplies like a backpack and footwear. But after that, your daily costs are totally in your control. You can do it as cheaply—or as lavishly—as you would like.

In terms of accommodation, there is choice for every pocketbook. Albergues are the dorm-style accommodation with bunk beds and shared bathroom facilities. The municipal (or public) albergues are your cheapest option, with private albergues offering a few more amenities at a slightly higher cost. Private rooms in hostels or a casa rural are your next step up, and fancy hotels or retreat centres are on the high end. If you purchase a guidebook or download any Camino apps, they will be able to provide approximate, up-to-date costs and also more detail about lodging and specific amenities.

Same goes for food. The standard pilgrim meal (usually a meat, french fries, and salad) is often seen as the least expensive option, but you can also eat even more economically by buying your own food at a grocery store and cooking for yourself (or with a group of new friends!). Many albergues have shared kitchen facilities. And if money isn't tight, there are all kinds of cafés and restaurants, ranging all the way up to Michelin-starred.

Choices that may increase your overall costs are taking a taxi or a bus rather than walking, and having to purchase additional items that you didn't bring from home (e.g., bandages, ibuprofen, sunscreen, walking sticks, or additional clothing). That said, food and accommodation will be your two main costs, and you get to choose on a daily basis how much you spend.

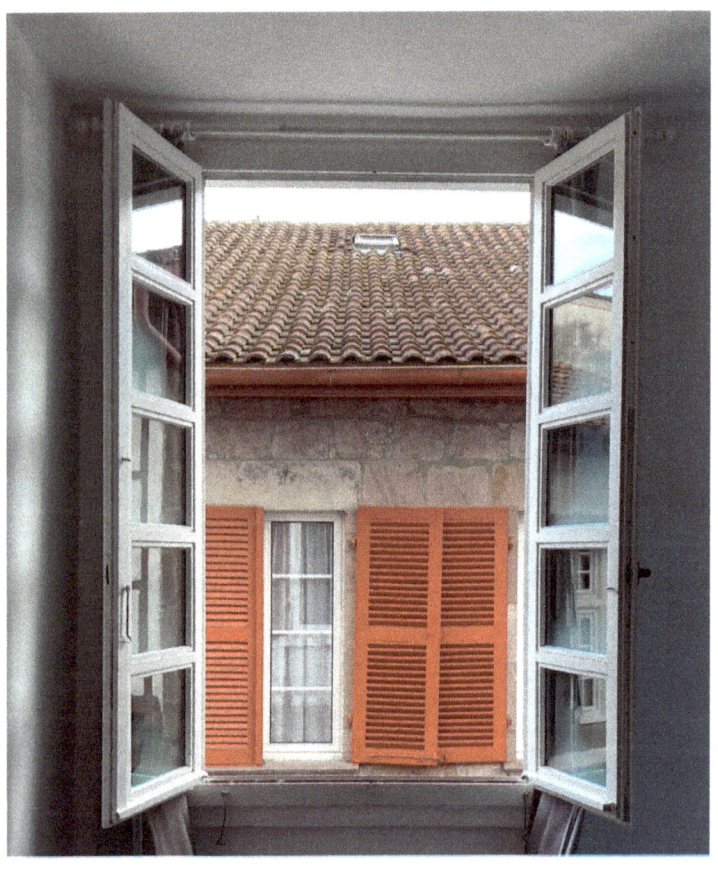

TIME

Being able to take a big chunk of time out of life or off work can be one of the biggest barriers when it comes to walking the Camino. This is especially true if you choose to traverse the Camino Francés from the traditional starting point of Saint-Jean-Pied-de-Port in France—it's no small feat at around 800 kilometres (500 miles).

I think this is why so many retired people are on the trail. They have the freedom of no longer working and can take their time. No need to hurry back. If this is you, you can enjoy a more leisurely trip.

If you are still working and have limited vacation time or are self-employed and need to be attentive to your business, taking more than a month off may be difficult. It doesn't mean you have to give up on your dream, though. Here are some options if you have limited time:

- You could consider doing only a single section of any of the Camino trails. I talked to scores of people who did this, many of them returning year after year to complete a subsequent section.

- You could also choose to do one of the shorter Camino routes. The Camino Ingles is around 100 km, the Camino Portuguese from Porto is 260 km, and the Camino Primitivo is 321 km.

- Traditionally, people who had less time at their disposal but still wanted to receive the Compostela certificate (a document given to pilgrims who meet the walking requirements) would walk the last 100 km from Sarria to Santiago. That's because the requirements used to state that in order to receive your Compostela, you needed to walk the *last* 100 km. However, in 2025 the rules changed! The requirements now say that you can walk *any* 100 km of any Camino but that you must walk the last "stage" into Santiago (from O Pedrouzo, roughly 20 km) in order to receive your Compostela certificate. This gives you more flexibility in terms of choosing the walk that is right for you. And it will also hopefully lead to less congestion on this final section of the Camino!

ARE YOU READY FOR YOUR WANDER?

When you walk the Camino alone, you are in charge of every aspect of your experience. You can fully focus on yourself and your own needs and desires, without having to worry about taking care of anyone else. You get to decide what you want to do, where you want to stay, and the time frame for everything. You come first. Every day of your Camino journey. Doesn't that sound freeing?

I hope the topics covered in this section have illuminated what might be holding you back and have made the idea of a big solo trip seem more doable. And just in case you need a little more encouragement, let this list of what I gained from my Camino act as a tipping point for you:

- Despite sore feet and a couple of blisters, my body was happy when I was walking. The life of a writer means sitting in one place for too long every day, and my body rejoiced in the constant motion of thirty-five days spent walking. I lost my ordinary aches and pains and generally felt looser. I discovered first-hand that movement is indeed medicine, and yes, motion is lotion.

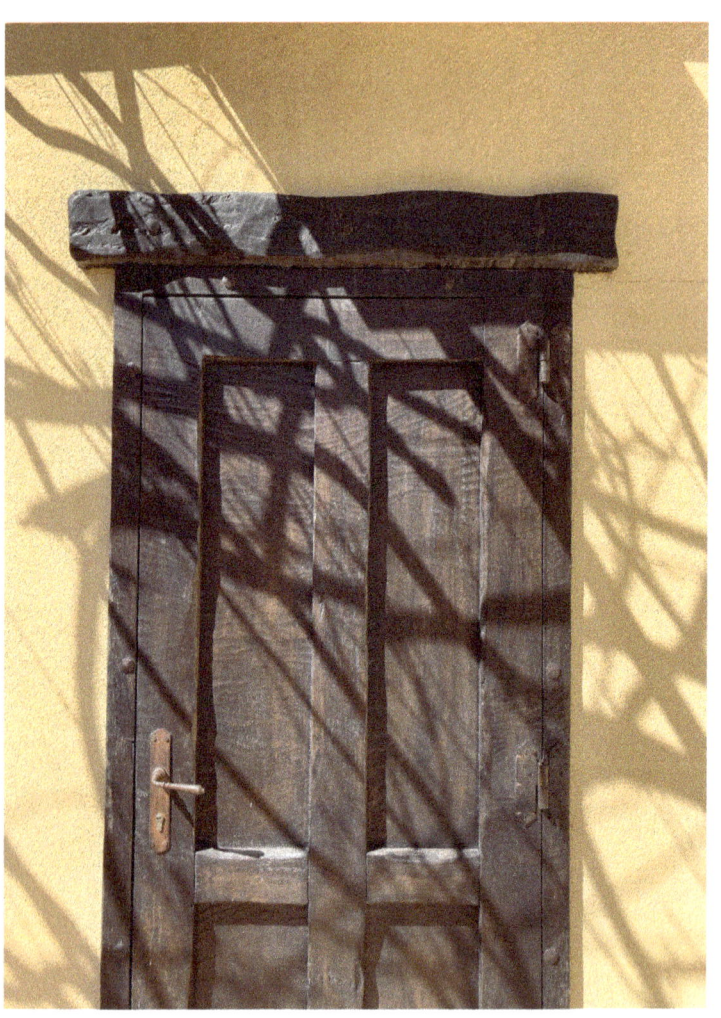

- I loved being outside for so much of every day, passing through different landscapes and having my feet on the earth and my ears attuned to the sounds of nature.

- The Camino is, by its very nature, a simple thing to do. You put one foot in front of the other, and you walk. I loved this simplicity—both in terms of what I was carrying with me and what was expected of me. My life at home is busy, so enjoying six weeks of a greatly reduced to-do list felt liberating. The regular tasks and requirements of life fell away, and I was left with the most basic "survival" requirements: walk to my next destination, find food to eat, and secure a place to sleep.

- This simplicity led to a slowing down internally, as if my nervous system was being reset. I thought a lot about how, in "regular life," we are bombarded with so much distraction and sometimes dragged from our core selves by the loud and insistent voices of a culture that doesn't necessarily align with who we really are.

- I definitely discovered new things about myself, and I had the spaciousness to reflect on what I was learning.

- I felt stronger and more resilient when I finished the Camino. I also felt more comfortable in my own skin, more confident making decisions on my own behalf, and proud of myself.

I hope you are feeling more aware of the things that might be holding you back and also maybe a bit more confident about moving ahead. If so, the rest of the book is intended to help you prepare for and enjoy your journey.

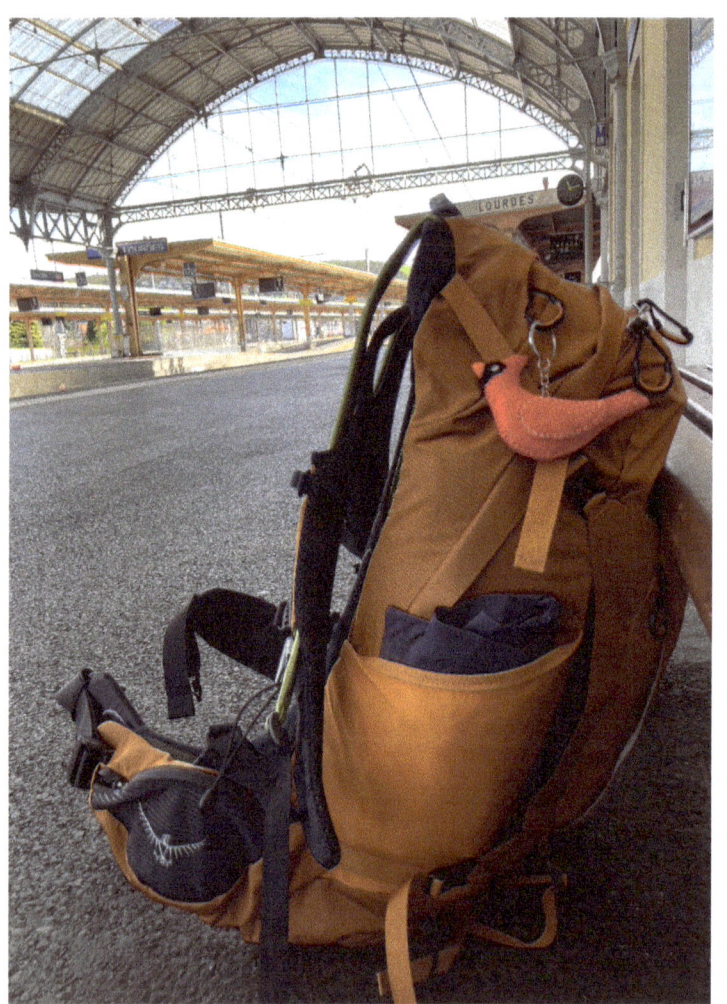

PART TWO

CHOOSE YOUR PATH AND PACK YOUR BAG

When you choose to walk the Camino on your own, you're in for a real adventure, one that begins as soon as you start preparing. Setting a date, buying a plane ticket, researching, training, and packing your bag are all important parts of getting ready for your big solo trip.

This section will cover the physical, mental, and emotional aspects of preparing to walk your Solo Camino.

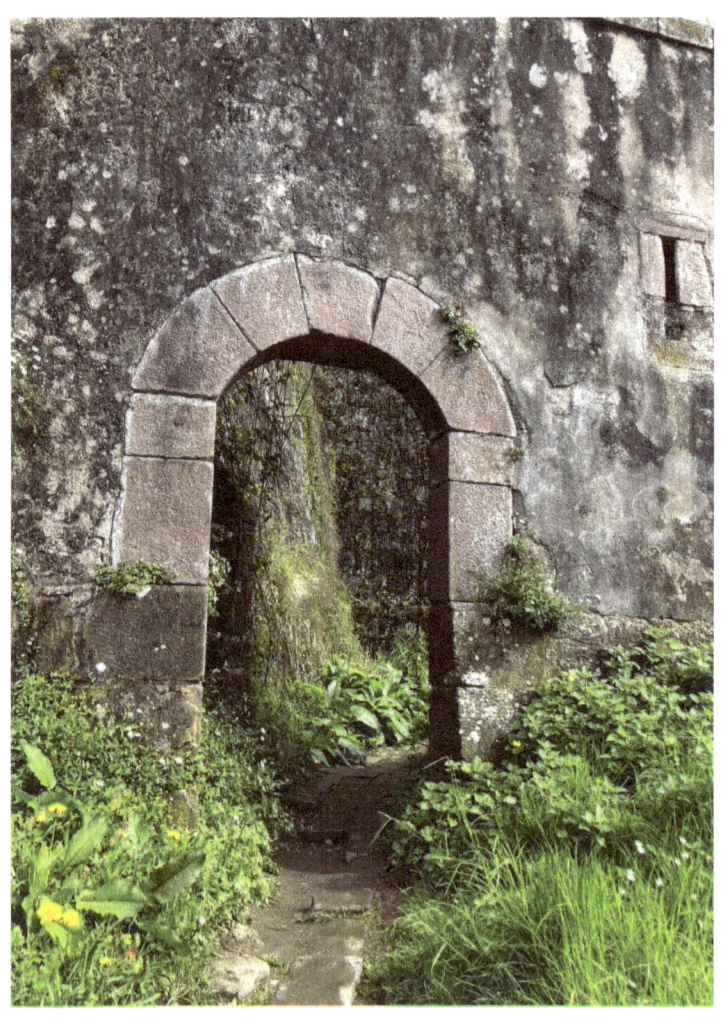

DISCOVER YOUR WHY

"Why are you doing the Camino? What do you hope to get out of it?"

I was asked things like this many times before I left for Spain. The truth is that I really struggled to answer those questions, partly because there wasn't one specific explanation.

I was drawn to the physical challenge. I had a longing for simplicity. And there was an undeniable itch to have a real adventure. I also hoped to make new friends from around the world, see beautiful cities and countryside, and explore my own spirituality.

It wasn't just one thing. But in the weeks leading up to the trip, when I really thought and wrote about it, a fresh clarity surfaced and there was a whisper of a new answer there: "I want to learn to trust myself. I want to feel I am providing my own sense of safety."

I was raised in a family with a protective father who was focused on keeping his children safe. The doors were always locked. The stove was checked before we went out. And there were strict rules about strangers and accepting rides and always calling to say you had gotten to your destination safely.

As a parent now myself, I know he felt it was his job to protect my sister and me from all manner of disaster and mayhem.

But I was already an anxious kid, and my dad's hypervigilance caused me to become even more worried. And that fear and anxiety never really left me, even as a grown woman walking through the world.

In fact, in my whole life, I had never taken a solo trip.

When I searched my heart, what I hoped for was a chance to trust myself and keep myself safe, without anyone else there to look after or support me. I wanted to be able to proclaim that I had taken a trip alone—and that I had succeeded.

REFLECTION / WRITING PROMPTS:

What is your WHY? What do you hope to get out of walking the Camino alone?

Is there something obvious and concrete you are hoping to achieve? Or is there a whisper of an answer, like I had?

SET YOUR OWN INTENTIONS

When you walk the Camino, because it is an ancient pilgrimage route, you will be referred to as a pilgrim or peregrina (female pilgrim in Spanish). But what does this mean, and more specifically, what does it mean to you?

I want to tell you something that I wish someone had told me. Something I wish I'd known during my own planning process. **There is no one right way to do the Camino.**

There is a lot of information out there about what pilgrims are and are not, and what they should do and not do. If you've done any amount of research via books or videos or websites, you'll have seen some of these "Camino Rules" on display. For instance, "Pilgrims are supposed to carry their knapsacks the whole way," or "If you don't walk every step, you didn't really do the Camino," or "You're not a real pilgrim if you don't sleep in albergues every night," or "Real pilgrims don't listen to music while walking." Hmmm.

I would like to think that on a pilgrimage route like the Camino, people would be allowed to do their own thing without judgment or censorship, but these "rules" can still get in our heads. If you enter into your Camino like I did, without questioning these rules and figuring out if they resonate with you, you are setting yourself up for shame and guilt when you actually want or need something different or when something goes awry.

I want to advise you to set your own intentions about how you want your trip to unfold. And to make your own personal commitments about this journey. What does it mean FOR YOU to be a pilgrim? How do YOU want to do this trip?

A wise person I met on the path gave me a mantra that I ended up repeating to myself many times along the way in many different circumstances: "The only rule about the Camino is that there are no rules." I found this enormously helpful, and I hope you do too.

This Camino you are preparing for is yours, and you can do it any way that feels right and best for you.

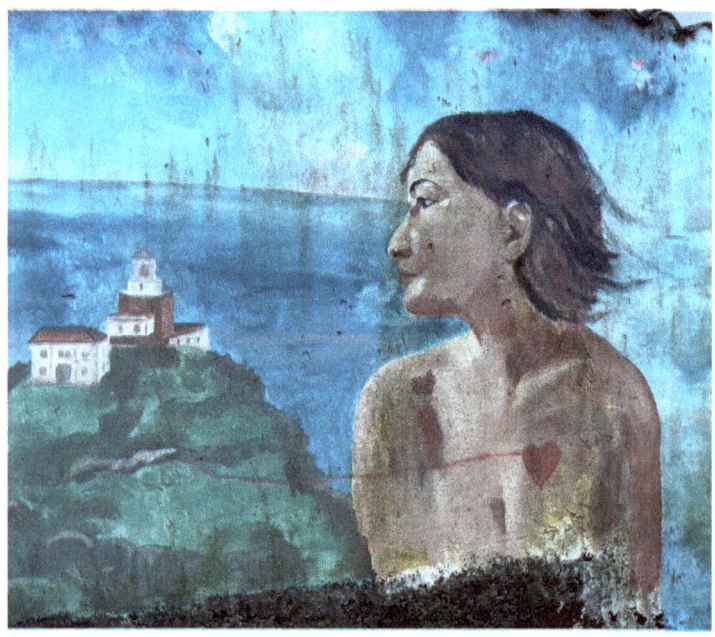

SET YOUR OWN INTENTIONS

REFLECTION / WRITING PROMPTS:

Here are a few questions that I wish someone had asked me to think about prior to walking the Camino:

Is it important for you to carry your own bag the entire way? If so, why? Is it because other people have said that's what a pilgrim does on the Camino, or do you have your own individual reason?

Do you intend to walk every step of the way, or are you open to taking a bus or a taxi if you need help for any reason?

Do you want to start your Camino in one of the traditional starting places, or is there another place that feels right to you and is more convenient?

Where do you want to sleep? Do you want to be in albergues with other pilgrims, or do you want to have a room of your own? Or maybe a mix?

Do you prefer walking with music or podcasts, or do you like silence? Or perhaps a bit of both?

How much socializing would you ideally like? How much alone time do you feel you may need?

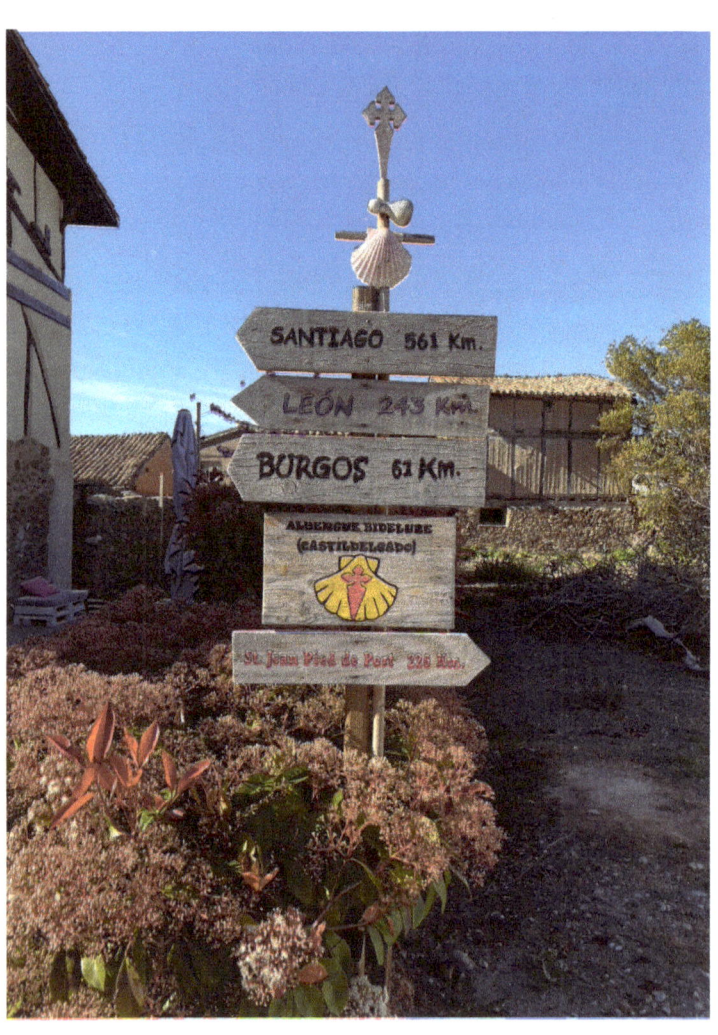

MAKE YOUR BIG DECISIONS

It's your Camino, and you get to decide what kind of trip you want to have. This means you choose which Camino route, what time of year you will walk, and what kind of experience you want to have.

WHICH ROUTE?

The Camino Francés, stretching from Saint-Jean-Pied-de-Port in France to Santiago de Compostela in Spain, is the route that most people think of as "the Camino," but there are actually 281 Camino routes through 29 different European countries covering over 8,000 km! Lots of choices!

Depending on how much time you have, which countries you want to pass through, and what kind of scenery you'd like to take in, you may want to consider another route.

I've met and talked to people who have done the Camino Portuguese, the Camino del Norte, the Camino Primitivo, and the Camino Ignacian. If you don't know about any of these paths, start researching!

As I mentioned in Part One, some of these routes are significantly shorter than the Camino Francés, so if you have less time available for your walk, one of the shorter Caminos may suit you better.

Many women who are first-time walkers choose to do the Camino Francés because of the built-up pilgrim infrastructure plus the large number of other walkers. When I was deciding which Camino to do, this one felt the safest and the easiest for me. After having successfully completed the Camino Francés, I would feel more confident tackling a quieter, less populated route the next time.

WHAT TIME OF YEAR?

The most popular months to walk the Camino are July and August, but that's also the hottest time. Many experienced pilgrims say the best months are May, June, and September for cooler temperatures, less rain, and fewer crowds.

Having walked in the spring, I can tell you that even in April and May, there is the potential for heat, downpours, and throngs of people. But it's also a gorgeous time of year, with so much new growth and life in the form of spring flowers, birdsong, and flowering trees.

My friends who have walked in the fall say they loved the crisp air, the grape harvest, and the autumnal colours in the forests.

It's up to you!

WHAT KIND OF AN EXPERIENCE?

In the book world, writers are either "plotters" or "pantsers." Plotters plan out the entire structure of their book from the first chapter to the last before they begin. Pantsers just start writing and see what happens (flying by the seat of their *pants*—get it?).

The Camino is the same, and I met both plotters and pantsers along the way. I also met people (myself included) who did a little bit of both. There is something reassuring about knowing where you are going to spend the night, but there is also something freeing about knowing you can stop whenever you want.

Here are a few different examples of possible Camino experiences:

Go-with-the-flow. For those who have a rough idea of where they want to end up at the end of a given day and the number of kilometres they want to cover but don't have any set plans and don't book any accommodation ahead of time.

Book in advance. For those who want the security of knowing where they will sleep on any given night. I usually did this one or two days ahead of time. It helped me to relax while I was walking, knowing I did not have to hurry in order to secure a bed. If you are a tried-and-true "plotter," you might be tempted to book all your days in advance, but I would caution against that, as it leaves absolutely no wiggle room. Do your research and find out if there are any stops on your Camino that may fill up fast (for example, if you are walking the Camino Francés and want to stop midway between Saint-Jean-Pied-de-Port and Roncesvalles on the first day, there are only a few options, and you may need to book weeks or months in advance).

Hire a company. I talked to women who were travelling solo but had hired a company to map out their route and book all of their accommodation. They walked roughly the same number of kilometres each day and didn't have to spend *any* time figuring out where to stay.

Go with a tour group. This option isn't technically a "solo" Camino, as you'll be moving from one place to another with others, but for some women it's a good starting place. One of my good friends did this and enjoyed having her bag transported and all accommodation and meals taken care of. These perks were part of the entry price. All she had to do was wake up and walk every day!

One thing to be aware of: the Camino Francés seems to be getting busier with each passing year. There were a number of times on my walk when, even though I was there in the "shoulder season" of April and early May, it took a significant amount of research, phone calls, and texting to be able to find a place to sleep, especially when looking for a private room.

BOOK YOUR PLANES AND TRAINS

For those who don't already live in Europe and need to fly there, I would recommend landing in London or Paris or Madrid and then taking either a short flight (using one of the budget airlines) or the train to your Camino starting point.

If you're walking the Camino Francés, Saint-Jean-Pied-de-Port is the best known and most used starting point for that route, but that doesn't mean that's where *you* need to start. I talked to all kinds of people who started their Camino in various other spots on the path: Roncesvalles, Pamplona, Logroño, Burgos, or Sarria. It really depends on how long a walk you have decided to take.

Here are some tips (some of which I learned the hard way!):

- Airfare and hotels can be more expensive if you travel on traditional holidays. I made the mistake of arriving in Europe on Easter weekend without having done the research that would have indicated that Easter is a huge holiday in Spain. Whoops!

- The budget airlines in Europe are sometimes cheaper than taking the train, especially those departing from England.

- Keep an eye on your long-haul flight four to six months in advance. I ended up getting quite a good price in December (right before Christmas too!) for a late March departure. Also, some savvy travellers I know sign up for Google Flights and are notified when their dream flight suddenly drops in price.

- If you can be flexible with your departure date and can fly out any day of the week, you may luck into a cheaper ticket on a Monday or Tuesday rather than a Saturday or Sunday.

- If you don't fly right to Spain, I would highly recommend you take the train through France for at least part of your journey. It's such a wonderful way to travel and is pretty economical.

- Consider building in a few days of rest and relaxation before your walk. Especially if you've travelled from overseas, it's helpful to have a day or two to acclimatize and get over jet lag before you start walking.

I envied people from Europe who didn't need to book a return flight home due to the ease and economy of travel within their own continent. Not having a firm end date is definitely an ideal scenario but is hard for many people to do.

GET YOUR BODY READY

And now for the fun part—getting your body ready!

Some people train so they are ready to walk twenty or thirty-kilometre days in a row with their backpack on (and even *train* with their pack fully loaded), while others don't train at all! My preparation fell somewhere in the middle. I gradually built up endurance in my daily walks and started going for longer hikes. I bought a watch to keep track of my steps, and I added some weight training to my health regimen. And for the last month before I left, I walked with my backpack and in the footwear I was taking (more on this in an upcoming chapter).

I also signed up for an organized long-form hike where we covered one hundred kilometres over five days and slept in church basements and community centres along the way. This was helpful to get a feel for what long walking days back to back would feel like. If you have time, and something like this is offered in the place you live, I would recommend it as a way to build your confidence and demystify the act of walking long distances.

WHAT WILL YOUR PHYSICAL PREPARATION TO WALK THE CAMINO LOOK LIKE?

If you are someone who doesn't move very much, but you long to be more active, it's good to start small and gradually build up your walking stamina. You don't have to go from 0 to 100 immediately; simply begin by incorporating walking into your daily routine and then slowly increase your distances.

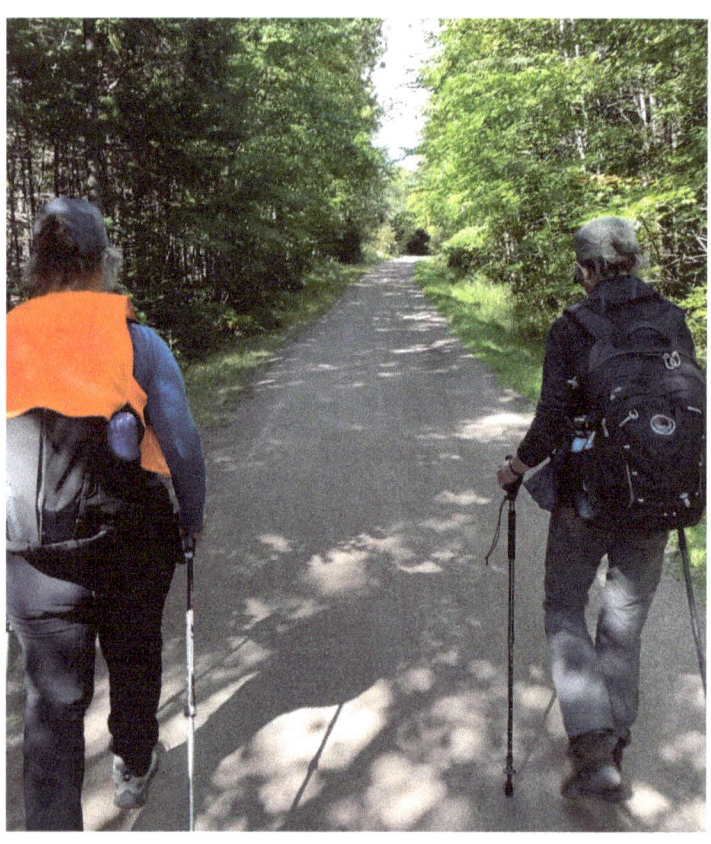

Once you are feeling more confident and a bit stronger, that's the time to consider investing in a piece of equipment like a watch that tracks your steps. It will likely help with your focus and your commitment to your walking habit.

On the flip side, if you are a fit person and walking is already a part of your daily routine, you won't have to train as much as someone who currently walks very little. That said, there is a big difference between walking ten thousand steps a day and walking twenty or more kilometres per day, many days in a row. Our bodies respond differently to long walking days, and we start to hurt in different places! My biggest piece of advice is to make time to go on longer walks and hikes, and keep building both your stamina and your distances.

REFLECTION / WRITING PROMPTS:

Here are a few factors to consider and a few questions to ask yourself:

What kind of shape are you are currently in?

How much walking do you regularly do?

Have you done anything like this before?

Do you have appropriate footwear for longer walks?

Do you have any health conditions or body limitations? If so, what kind of support can you set up for yourself?

Can you make a plan to increase the distances you are walking?

What are some ways you can support your physical training (e.g., buy good shoes, find an accountability buddy, join a walking club, buy a fitness tracker)?

PLAN AND RESEARCH

Back in the day, if you wanted to do the Camino, you bought a guidebook, packed a backpack, and off you went. Nowadays, you could honestly spend years researching and planning your trip—that's how much information is out there!

If you have a tendency toward overthinking, overplanning, and procrastination, be aware! It's easy to get overwhelmed by the volume of tips and advice, which could lead to getting stuck in planning mode. My advice would be to do some research but move quickly into the action phase, trusting yourself to figure it out.

Here is a short list of what types of Camino resources are out there:

Books. As you probably know, no shortage of books have been written about the Camino. There are memoirs of first-hand experiences, and there are books about specific aspects of the Camino—culinary adventures, sacred sites, plus bird and plant guides. There are books written with the sole purpose of helping you pack the right items and walk without getting blisters. And then, of course, there are the guidebooks with maps, distances, lists of accommodations, and information about local history. These are usually slim and many people bring one along to consult as they walk.

Movies/Videos. While *The Way* is probably the most well-known of the Camino movies, there are lots of films and documentaries to explore. There are also endless YouTube videos documenting people's personal journeys.

Websites/Blogs. There are so many of these that it's honestly a little overwhelming. In my mind, the best Camino websites are the ones where you don't feel inundated with advertising and that answer some of your most basic questions. There are also some amazing Camino blogs with photos and diary entries if you want to read about someone else's daily routines and experiences.

Forums. These are online sites with thousands of members where you can post questions and receive helpful information. If you type a question such as "Which backpack for the Camino" or "Best shoes for walking" or "Do I need to book a bed ahead of time," some of your most prominent search results will likely come from forums like these. They are usually free to join, as long as you don't mind being served up ads (always for Camino-related purchases).

Facebook Groups. There are a number of groups on Facebook that are geared toward women walking the Camino. You can post questions and receive answers from women who have walked before. You can also potentially connect with other women who might be starting their Camino around the same time as you, if you feel nervous beginning your trip alone.

PLAN AND RESEARCH

Podcasts. There are a few podcasts that are solely about the Camino and the people who walk it. It's a great way to hear first-person accounts. If you've got a phone and some handy earbuds or headphones, you can listen while walking—training plus learning, all in one!

Camino Associations. These exist to help people connect with others in their own regions or countries who have walked—or hope to walk—the Camino. They may organize local hikes, have meet-and-greets, offer information, and sell the Camino passport or credential that you will need to get stamped on a daily basis if you hope to receive your certificate of completion (Compostela) in Santiago.

In addition to information about packing, getting there, where to stay, etc., make sure you also do a little research on the country itself—history, customs, food. You don't want to be one of those tourists who is so focused on walking that you don't respect or appreciate the country you are passing through.

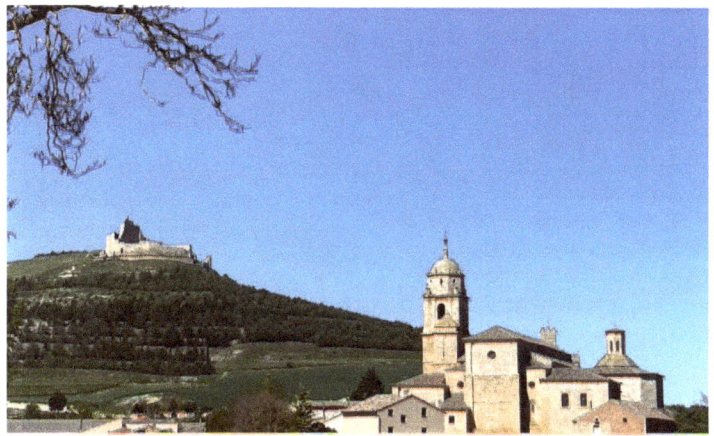

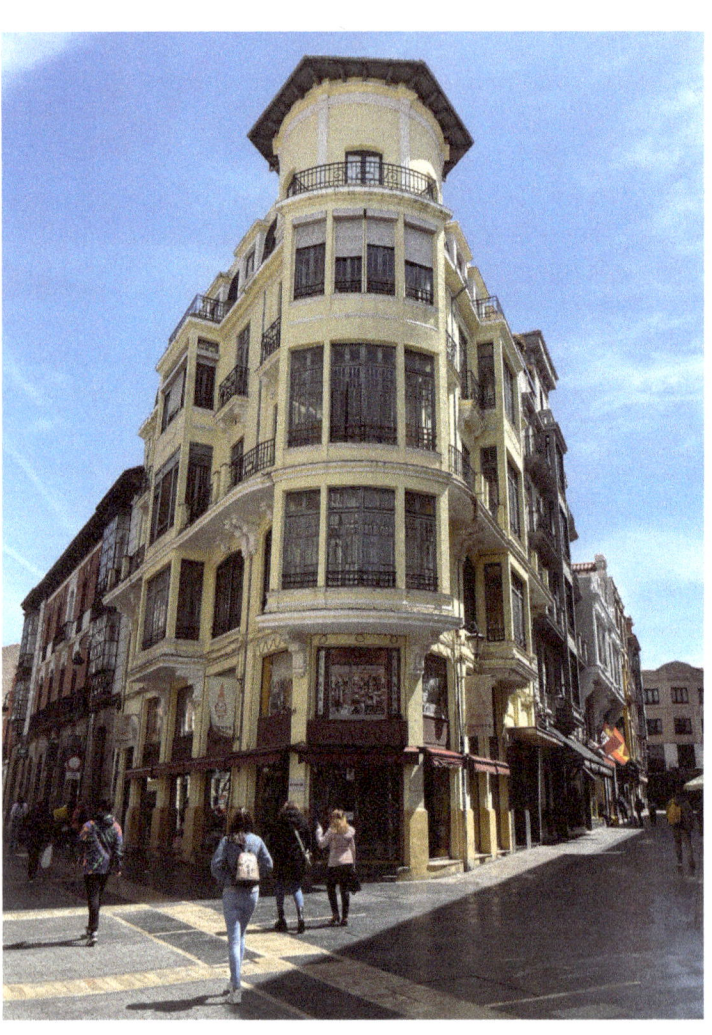

LEARN THE LANGUAGE

When the Camino became a reality for me—as in, *I'm really going to do this*—I bought a one-year membership to the online language tool Duolingo. This was helpful when it came to learning vocabulary, but for me, it wasn't a good way to learn how to actually converse in Spanish.

So, a few months before my trip began, I signed up for a Spanish language course that was specific to the Camino. My Spanish teacher lived right on the Camino in Spain, and we had weekly video calls where she helped me learn and practise specific phrases I would need. This was enormously helpful and something I highly recommend.

When you walk the Camino, there are precise vocabulary phrases you need to learn to be able to ask for what you need. For instance: a bed, a room, a blanket, a coffee or tea, a piece of toast. You should also know how to say hello, goodbye, please and thank you, and help me.

Please don't assume that every Spanish person who happens to live on the Camino speaks English (many don't). And please don't be someone who decides, out of ignorance or fear, to not learn any Spanish at all. The courteous and kind thing to do is to attempt to speak the language of the country you are in. You don't have to be fluent, but I believe it is important to try—and people will usually appreciate your attempt!

On that note, my Spanish teacher gave me a very important piece of advice. She said that in Spain the most important thing—even more important than saying please and thank you—is to greet the person you are about to attempt conversation with. Look them in the eye, smile, say hello, and perhaps even ask how they are doing (in Spanish, of course). It's a demonstration of cultural respect.

In my experience, the people of Spain appreciate pilgrims who attempt to order food or reserve a room in Spanish. They are also, for the most part, very kind and helpful. If they see you trying to speak Spanish (and maybe humorously failing), and if they do happen to know English, many will switch over to relieve you of your fumbles! They will also definitely be more accommodating toward you because you gave it a shot.

In addition to taking a course, consider listening to one of the many Spanish-language podcasts or watching short Spanish videos (some of these are geared to beginners).

PACK YOUR BAG

As I mentioned earlier, one of the great things about the Camino is its simplicity. In a world that encourages us, at every turn, to buy and consume *more*, it's really refreshing to have the emphasis shift to *less*.

You walk with a simple backpack containing the bare essentials and no frills. This may feel quite different to other trips you've been on, where your suitcase is stuffed with "just in case" items and lots of choice in terms of footwear and clothing. This is a much simpler journey and a lighter way of life.

When it comes to your packing list, keep that focus on simplicity front and centre. Don't buy into the notion that you need a bunch of fancy gadgets or that you have to buy all new items or all brand name items. Use stuff that you already have, and check out second-hand stores too. This will make it more affordable to splurge on a few new items that you might really need (good hiking shoes, a comfortable backpack, etc.).

There are entire books, and long videos on YouTube, devoted to what to pack for your Camino, so I am not going to reinvent the wheel here. If you *are* interested in my packing list, go to the Camino tab on my website (reneehartleib.com) where I've made some resources available.

Your packing list will depend on which route you've chosen, how long you are going to be away, and what kind of a trip you've decided on. For instance, if you already know that your goal is to carry your own bag, weight will become your number one priority.

There is a "Camino rule" that your bag shouldn't be more than 10 percent of your body weight, but this can cause a lot of angst for small people (it's hard to have only a five-kilogram pack) and trouble for larger people (who probably shouldn't carry eleven to twelve kilograms just because it's technically 10 percent of their weight).

The truth is that you can train to carry more than 10 percent of your body weight—if you need everything in that bag. But do you? Remember: Spain is a country where you will be able to find anything and everything you need, usually within a day or two. If something on your packing list is a "maybe," consider leaving it at home, knowing you can pick it up when you get there (if you decide it's really necessary!).

Here are my top pieces of advice when it comes to packing for the Camino. I've tried to keep this list short and to include things you may not have read about or heard elsewhere.

Pack a thin piece of foam for sitting. I repurposed a gardening pad from home, intended for kneeling, that was slender and foldable. Every time I needed to stop and sit, air out my shoes, or have a snack, I pulled it out. Having a soft cushion between my bum and rocks, logs, or hard benches felt like a little piece of heaven. When other women saw me using this little foam pad, they inevitably said, "So smart!"

Bring or buy a rain poncho. I originally thought that a raincoat would suffice but at the last minute bought a poncho in Saint-Jean-Pied-de-Port. So glad I did! It kept me and my bag dry on the wettest of days. If you are worried about being wet and cold, see my chapter on the inevitable rain of Galicia in Part Three for more tips!

PACK YOUR BAG

Bring your own ibuprofen and sunscreen. I found both of these items to be more expensive in Spain, especially if you buy from a pharmacy (farmacia) as opposed to the pharmacy section of a large grocery store.

Use a belt bag for your phone, passport, pilgrim credential, money, lip balm, tissues, etc. It saves you from having to take off your backpack and root around for what you need.

Buy a recyclable plastic water bottle from a store en route, rather than bringing your own water bottle. It's lighter and you also won't be sad if you mistakenly leave it behind somewhere. I bought one of these—the kind with an easy "sports cap" nozzle rather than a screw top—at an airport store in my home city before boarding the plane, and it lasted for my entire trip!

Reusable bags and utensils. Bring your own reusable grocery bag for shopping and some zip-lock bags to keep leftovers fresh. Add in a "spork" and lightweight knife for cutting cheese or fruit and eating yoghurt or cereal, and you're all set! If you're a backcountry camper, you may already have a lot of what you need.

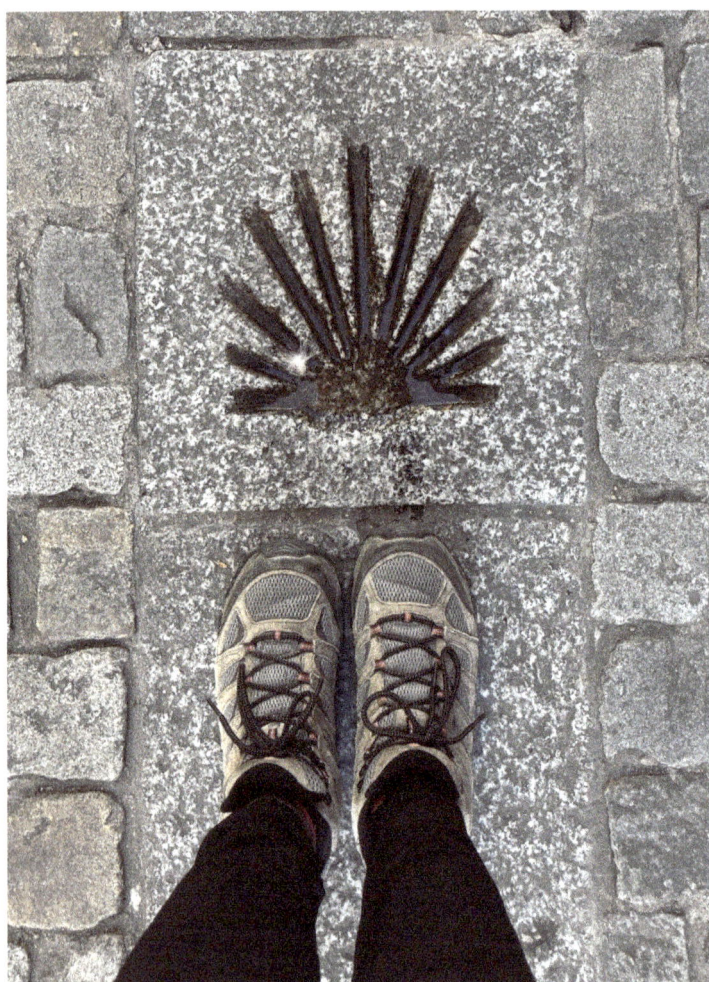

PREPARE YOUR FEET

I can't begin to tell you the number of pilgrims I met while walking the Camino who had debilitating blisters. These blisters were angry and infected and often altered the trajectory of people's journeys, causing them to seek medical attention, go on antibiotics, stop walking for days, and even cut their journey short.

It doesn't have to be like this! There are things you can do before your long-distance walk that will indicate which parts of your feet are prone to blisters. This allows you to plan accordingly.

First things first: footwear. What you wear on your feet is super important and also intensely personal. And there are lots of questions to ask yourself: A trail shoe or a boot? Waterproof or not? Lightweight or something with substance?

Finding a comfortable fit, when everyone's feet are so different, can be challenging. I literally spent months searching for the right footwear. All told, I bought and returned five or six different pairs of hiking boots. Each time, I wore them around the house and also walked at our local indoor track, and each time, there would be something not quite right. In the end, because my foot is wide, I opted for a men's version of a boot I liked, which worked out really well for me. In your own search, watch for spots that are too tight or that rub the wrong way, and give your feet lots of space to breathe. Don't settle for anything less than perfect!

Once I had chosen the best footwear for me, I turned my mind to blisters—a topic that showed up a lot in my research—and bought what I thought were the "best" blister bandages. I bought all different sizes and shapes for different parts of my feet. Turns out that was basically forty dollars down the drain.

Why? Because I only developed two blisters, both on my toes, and didn't end up needing the ones designed for other parts of the foot. The best remedy for my blisters ended up being inexpensive bandages I bought in the pharmacy section of a grocery store in Spain.

If I had done what I am about to suggest, I would have known where my blister-prone areas were and simply brought along a box of good old-fashioned Band-Aids!

Here it is, one of my biggest pieces of advice before you walk the Camino:

Set aside the time to do three or four days of back-to-back long walks with your fully loaded backpack and the shoes and socks you plan on walking in. If you are going to get blisters (and not everyone does!), I can guarantee you that three days of around twenty kilometres per day will clearly indicate your problem areas for blisters and give you a chance to play with what kind of blister care works best.

Here are a few other foot care tips that helped me:

- As you walk, if you feel a hot spot, a stone in your shoe, or something rubbing the wrong way, it's crucial that you stop and deal with it as soon as you notice. This might be annoying in the moment, but there is no point in pushing through; it will only bring misery for days.

PREPARE YOUR FEET

- Use a "body glide" lotion that helps protect your feet from friction and rubbing. I had a roll-on stick that I applied every morning before putting on socks and shoes.

- Wear merino wool socks that help keep feet drier and prevent blisters. When you stop to rest, take both shoes and socks off, giving your feet a chance to dry out. You could also consider changing your socks a few times a day, clipping the damp pair to your backpack to dry.

- Take along both a thin and a thick pair of socks. I ended up preferring my thin socks, as the thicker ones caused a heat rash on my feet. But when the weather got colder, I was happy for my thicker pair!

- Bring along a cream that contains arnica and rub it on your feet every night before sleep. I forgot to do this one night, and I really felt it the next day!

I met other pilgrims who had elaborate twenty-minute routines in the morning where they securely taped their feet to prevent blisters from forming. I didn't need to do this to avoid blisters, but if you decide it's needed once you start walking, there are literally hundreds of places on the Camino where you can buy foot care supplies. I found that the pharmacy sections of large grocery stores had a good selection of foot care products and were less expensive than what was available at farmacias.

Your feet are going to carry you through this journey from start to finish, and they need to be in good shape. Prepare ahead!

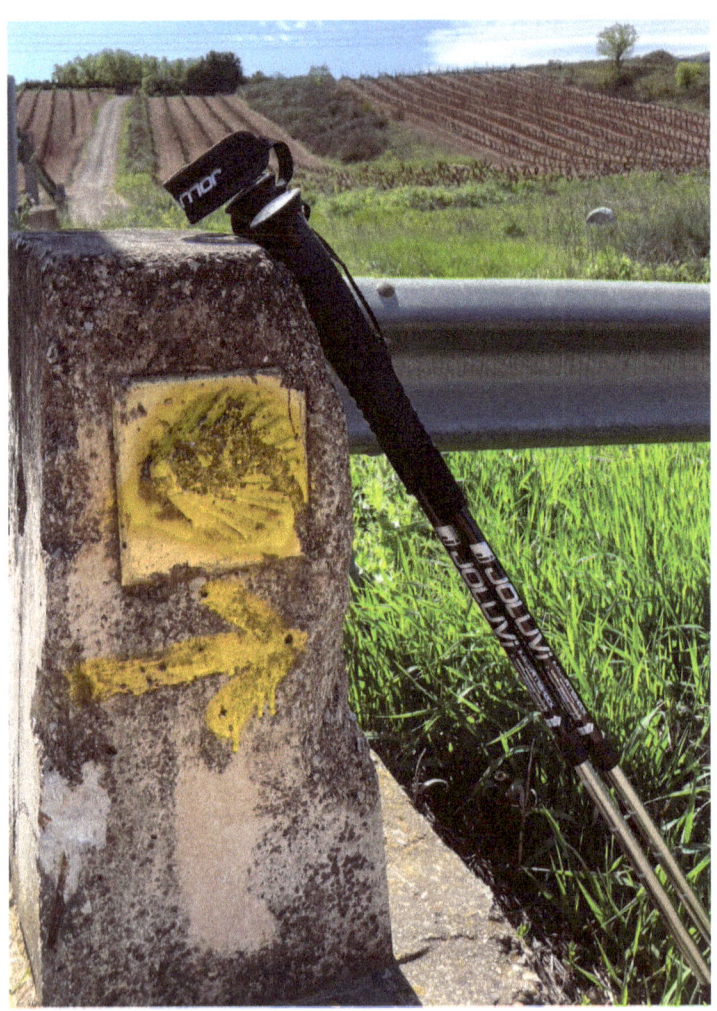

PICK YOUR POLES

Famous last words: "Well, I never use walking poles at home on our walks, so I don't know why I would use them in Spain." This is what I said to my partner in the weeks leading up to my departure date. "Yeah," she said, "I guess it must be personal preference."

We were both wrong. After having walked the Camino, I can say with absolute certainty that trekking poles (also called hiking poles or walking sticks) are enormously helpful with elevation, both up and down. They helped take strain off my knees, and they kept me more balanced. My daily walks at home had a few small hills, but nothing compared to the Camino. That's why I couldn't possibly know that I would actually need them.

Thank goodness the Camino has outfitter stores along the route! I was helped by a knowledgeable, multilingual shop owner in Pamplona who explained that I needed a good quality pole that would get me to Santiago, but not something top-of-the-line. Even though I was a trekking pole neophyte, he didn't try to upsell me, and I appreciated that.

If you plan ahead, you won't have to buy poles en route. But keep in mind that if you are carrying poles with you, airports all have different rules. Some will allow you through security if your poles are collapsible, while others don't allow any kind of pole at all. Look into the rules for the airports on your route. And if the price isn't out of your range, you could always consider checking a bag to avoid the risk of pole confiscation.

If you do end up having to buy poles once you're walking, try them out in the store and get advice on the correct length of pole for your height. If you buy adjustable ones, you can fold them up for sections of the path where you might not need them. And make sure you buy the rubber tips so you don't drive other walkers crazy with your tap, tap, tapping!

INVESTIGATE TECHNOLOGY

Ah, technology! The bane of our existence, or something you don't even want to imagine living without? We humans are divided on the steadily advancing pace of technology and constantly debate whether it enhances or detracts from our lives.

When it comes to the Camino, there are people who don't take *any* technology along—even a phone—although these are the rare pilgrims nowadays. Most folks, even if they aren't spending a lot of time on social media or consuming news, use their phones to take photos and to stay connected to family and friends.

If you are someone who is looking forward to a tech-free Camino, skip over this section. If you are interested in the technology available to Camino walkers, read on.

Phone. If you do bring your phone, I would suggest having it in airplane mode while you walk. That way your phone battery won't run down and die as it searches for cell service. You can still take photos when your phone is offline!

Other devices. Up to you. I saw people with e-readers, tablets, and even computers. For me, the extra weight wasn't worth it.

Earbuds/Headphones. For listening to music or a podcast as you walk, for having a conversation with family back home, or for drowning out snorers in an albergue, these are a great, lightweight idea.

Watch. It's fun to have a watch that calculates the number of steps per day. You'll be amazed! But don't fall into the trap of buying a super expensive one that has all the bells and whistles (especially if you don't learn how to use any of it!). A simple, good quality fitness tracker doesn't have to cost an arm and a leg. And if a watch doesn't appeal to you but you like the idea of tracking your steps, your phone should be able to do the job.

Charging Ports. You can charge your devices in most albergues, although there may be a crowd waiting to do the same thing. If you stay in a private room, you'll have your own outlet, and charging won't be an issue. Remember, you will need a European adapter for electrical plugs in Spain! I would also suggest bringing a small, lightweight power bank or portable charger for longer days. If your phone dies before you reach your destination, you can charge it while you are still walking.

Wi-Fi. There was free Wi-Fi available every place I stayed and often in cafés and restaurants along the route. This will enable you to touch base at home when needed, download a map, or email or text to find accommodation.

SIM Cards. I have good news for you. Having to buy a SIM card when you land in a foreign country and safely storing your own is a thing of the past. The modern-day equivalent is called an eSIM. You purchase it online and use your phone to activate it when you

INVESTIGATE TECHNOLOGY

get to your destination. No physical card required! I did quite a lot of research before I left and went with a well-reviewed company that offers service in Spain. I chose an eSIM with unlimited data that was a bit more expensive, but it meant I didn't have to worry about running out and having to top up my data plan. The peace of mind that came with being able to freely use my phone, in between towns or with no access to Wi-Fi, was well worth the extra cost! That said, I met people who didn't use an eSIM at all, totally relied on Wi-Fi, and they felt it was enough.

Camino Apps. There are a number of Camino apps you can download on your phone and that serve different purposes. Some offer maps and show you in real time if you are on or off the path (very helpful!). Others help plan your route, tell you the number of kilometres between towns, and give information about the area you're in. And still others offer accommodation options and reviews. I recommend you check out what other people have said about any albergues, hostels, or hotels you are considering. I found this so helpful in making decisions. And if you have a few minutes to help other pilgrims, don't forget to leave a review if you want to share the love about a certain special spot.

For more information on the specific names of some of the apps I used and the eSIM card I purchased, go to the Camino resources page of my website (reneehartleib.com).

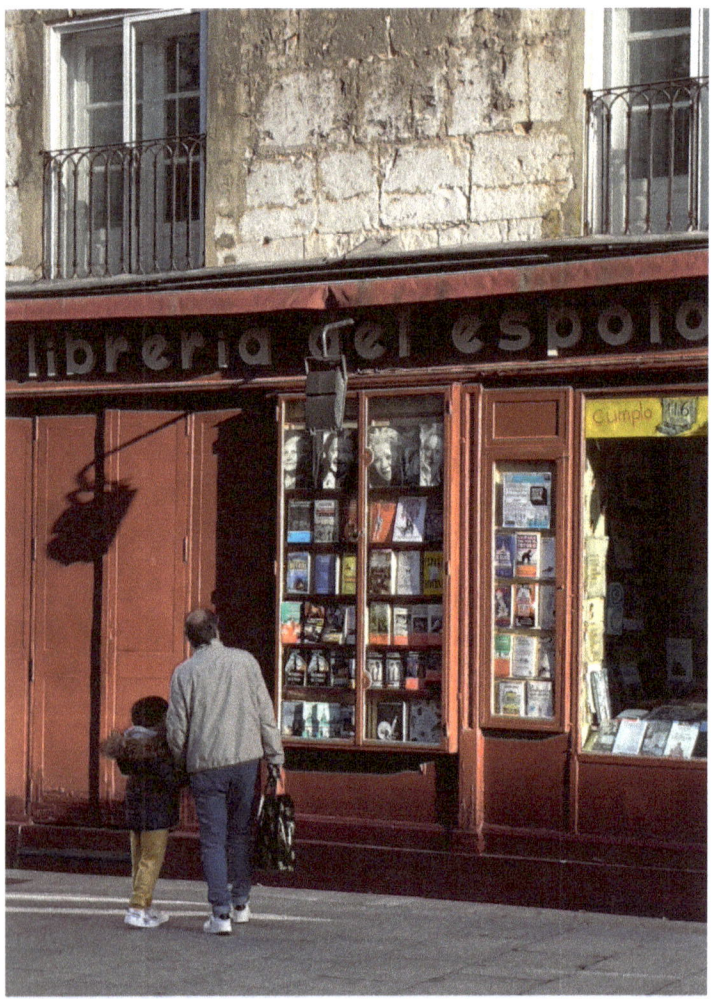

KEEP A JOURNAL

Even if you don't consider yourself a writer, I would highly recommend you take along a journal and try to write a little something each day.

Having done the Camino, I can tell you that when you get home and time passes, your days and your experiences and your memories will blend together. But if you're writing every day en route, you'll be able to record where you started each day, where you ended, and how many kilometres you walked. You'll also be able to note how you are feeling, jot down the names of people you meet, and write down any special experiences or insights you have.

Not only will an intentional practice like journalling assist you in remembering your trip once you return home, it also helps you make the most of this gift of time and this prolonged break from your usual life. I know I'm biased as a writer, but I strongly believe that writing encourages a deeper connection with ourselves. Writing things down helps make things real and has the power to provoke a change in mindset, attitude, or outlook. It also ensures that our good ideas and epiphanies don't get lost along the way.

Give it a try!

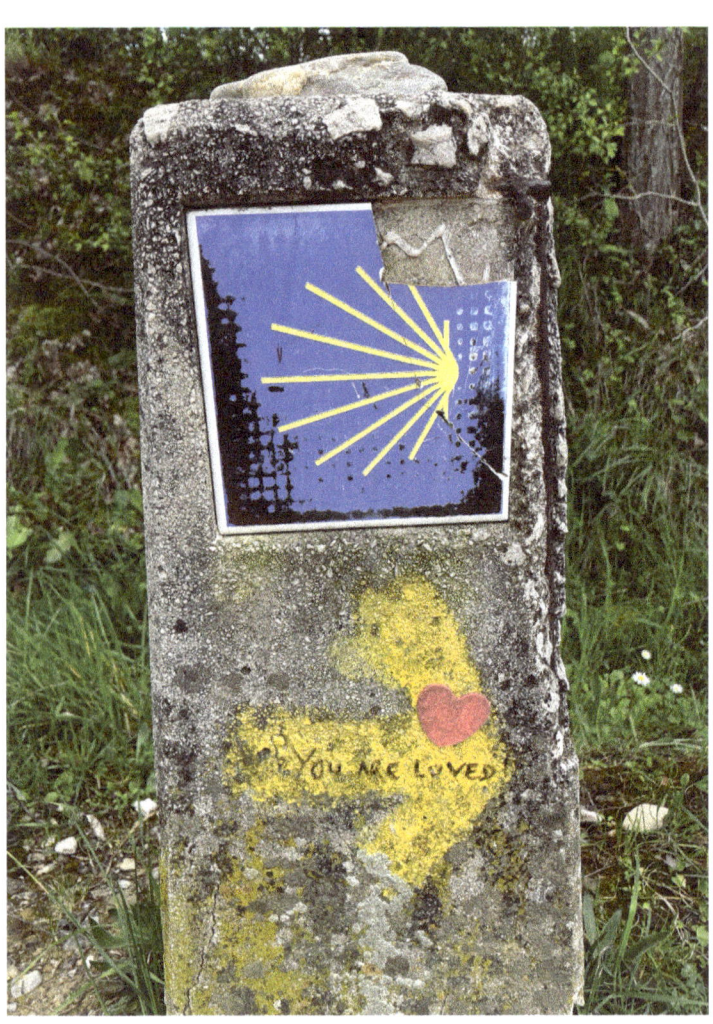

PART THREE

THE JOURNEY ITSELF: WHAT I LEARNED ON MY CAMINO

We've talked about what might be holding you back and what you can do to prepare. Now this section is all about the trip itself!

Wherever you choose to start and however long your walk, there are things all these journeys have in common: finding places to eat and sleep, physical and emotional challenges, connection with others. And sometimes, epiphanies or angst.

In this part of the book, I've included personal Camino stories from my trek along the Camino Francés, plus practical tips. I also make special mention of taking care of your body and spirit.

My hope is that these stories and my advice—split into The Beginning, The Middle, and The End—will give you the heads-up on what to expect, help you feel more prepared, and serve as inspiration for your own adventure ahead.

THE BEGINNING

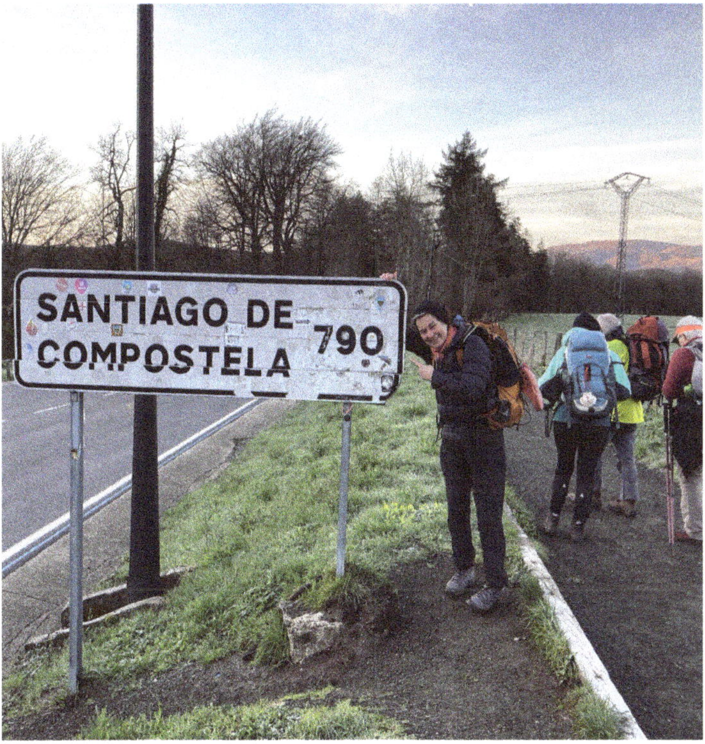

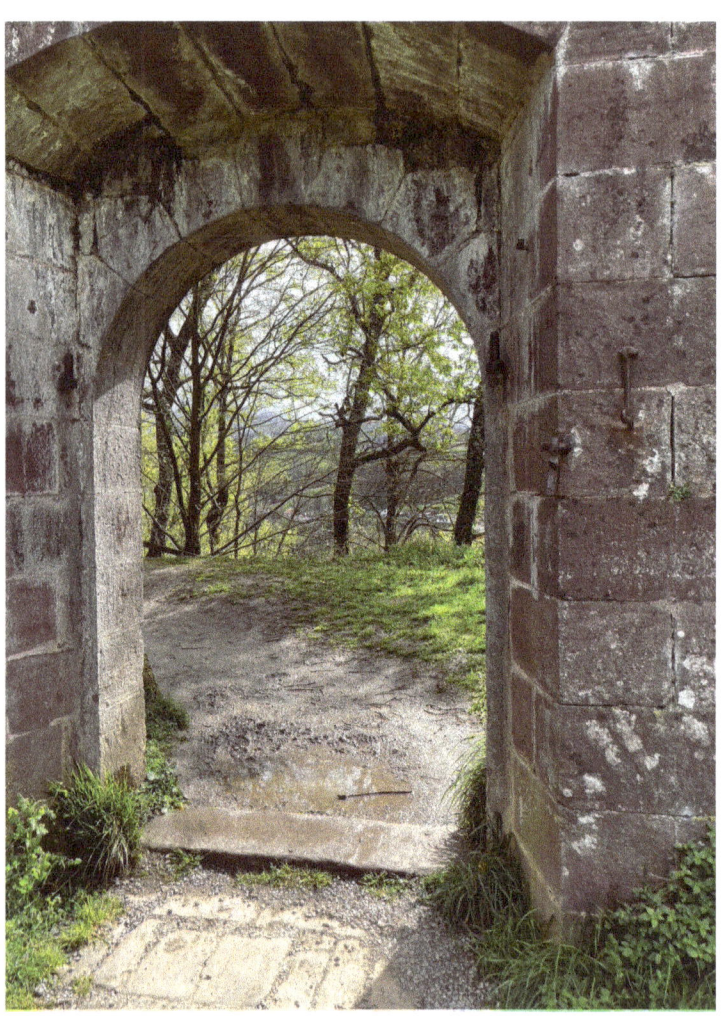

STEPPING OUT

I will never forget the feeling of my first few steps on the Camino.

It was April 1, 2024, in Saint-Jean-Pied-de-Port, the traditional starting place of the Camino Francés. I was staying in a beautiful sixteenth-century Basque home, called Gîte Beilari, run by the wonderful Joseph and Flor. The night before, around the supper table, I'd met people from many different countries—France, the Netherlands, Malaysia, Germany, Canada, and the United States. Joseph had asked us thought-provoking questions about the deep "why" of the journey we were about to embark on, and when we shared our answers over candlelight and Flor's delicious home-cooked meal, it brought a feeling of magic and intimacy to a table full of strangers.

On that first morning of the epic walk, I fuelled up with tea, toast, and a soft egg as the adrenalin surged through my body. I brushed my teeth, laced up my boots, gave goodbye hugs, hoisted my pack onto my back, and loitered a little, waiting for others to leave. I wanted to walk out that door alone. On this solo journey of mine, I felt like I needed to take the first steps of my Camino on my own.

When I did, the sky was just lightening, the air was cool and still, and the morning birds were singing. The large cobblestones held my feet the moment before I took a deep breath and stepped forward on the path.

Thank you, thank you, thank you. Those were the words I breathed out as my eyes filled with tears and I felt myself overflowing with gratitude. For my healthy body and also the unbelievable privilege of embarking on this kind of a journey, when it is simply not an option for so many.

These are my first steps on the Camino, I thought, tightening the straps of my backpack. These are my first steps of a very long road ahead. A road that will take me 800 kilometres from here, across the Pyrenees, and toward Roncesvalles, Pamplona, Burgos, and Leon, with hundreds of towns and villages in between, and finally to Santiago de Compostela.

Who will I be at the end of this journey? What will my final steps be like? Who are all the people I will meet? What are the experiences I will have?

When I look back on that first morning, I can still feel the joy of that moment and the freshness of my thoughts and energy.

I didn't know anything about the special people I would meet—a cheesemonger, an ultra-marathon runner, an Irish life coach, a British actress, an Instagram celebrity, a real estate mogul, a comedian, a plant biologist—and the vulnerable and moving conversations we would have. I didn't know that I would encounter lovely souls from some of the most war-torn countries in the world. I didn't know I would spend time with an order of singing nuns or be blessed in a tiny church outside of Burgos by another nun who looked me in the eyes and seemed to see into my soul.

I had no way of knowing all that was ahead: the heat wave that was coming ten days later; the sickness that felt endless; my own inner demons, who, upon seeing a blank open space, swooped in hard; the difficult decisions I would have to make; the terrible news I would receive from home.

In that moment, I was innocent to everything that would happen, the good, the not so good, and all the in-between. Despite the weight on my back, I felt as light as the shaft of sunlight that caught me as I passed through Porte Notre Dame and began the uphill climb toward Roncesvalles.

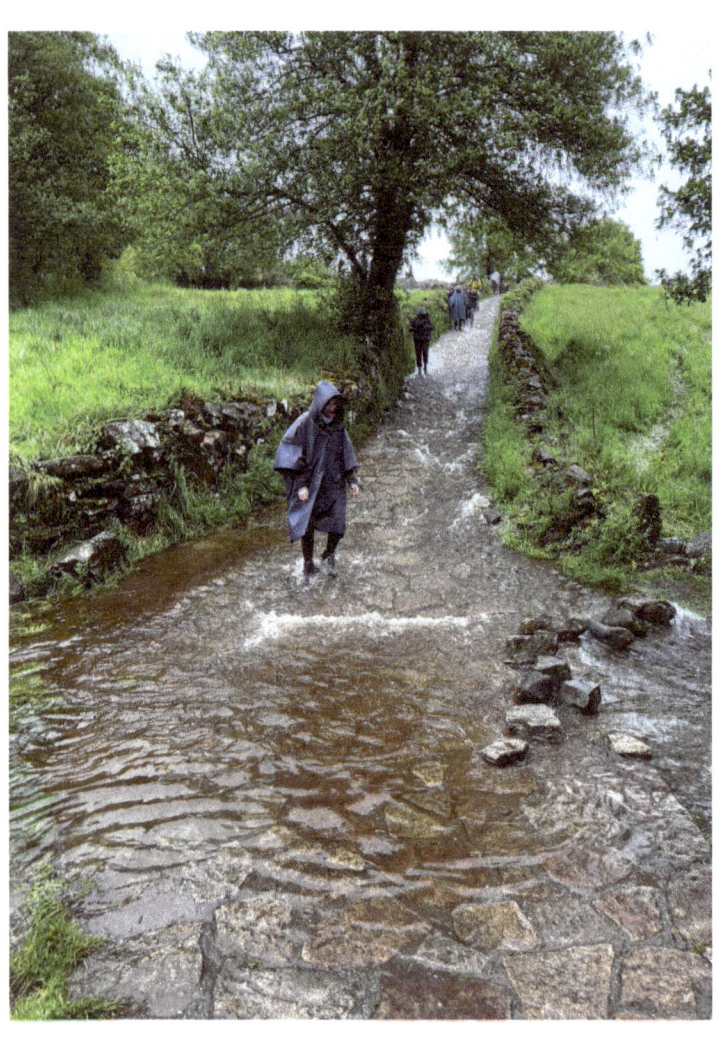

EXPECTING THE UNEXPECTED

There are two ways to get from Saint-Jean-Pied-de-Port to Roncesvalles: the Napoleon Route and the Valcarlos Route. The Napoleon is regarded as the more scenic, while the Valcarlos is referred to as the easier but less beautiful path. Both cross the Pyrenees, but the Napoleon has higher elevations and breathtaking *Sound of Music* vistas.

I had always imagined myself walking up and over the Pyrenees on a clear sunny day—my own "the hills are alive" moment—but the weather had other plans. The night before the Napoleon Route was set to open (April 1, the date many other pilgrims and I had built our trip around), I started hearing rumours. "It's snowing up there. It's pretty bad. I heard it's not going to open."

These rumours turned out to be true. The Napoleon Route stayed officially closed, and on April 1, I had to take that other path, the one I hadn't planned for or researched! Time to pivot and make the best of it, I thought, as I euphorically walked out of Saint Jean early that morning.

But by four p.m., long after the early lunch I'd had around eleven, I had not yet reached my destination, and the path was still angling upwards. I decided to take a break, ate some dried fruit and nuts, and remembered the wise advice of another pilgrim: "Take your socks and shoes off when you stop for snacks!" This person had even advised changing socks at least once per day.

I peeled off my socks to discover the start of a pretty massive blister on one of my toes. Oh no! And just as I was trying to dig out one of my fancy blister bandages, the sky, which had been gradually darkening, opened up. I shoved my feet back into my socks and shoes and hauled out the rain poncho I'd just bought in Saint Jean, struggling to figure out how to put it on.

An eternity later, I was walking again, scrambling up the now muddy path in a steep ascent. I began to hear an odd thudding in the trees above me and looked up to see enormous hailstones pelting down on me and all the pilgrims in front and behind me. A chorus of both excited whoops and anguished shouts erupted as I pulled out my phone to take a photo, only to have it die as I lifted it aloft to the sky.

There I was, about as far away as I could have imagined from my *Sound of Music* moment. Instead of sun, I had hail. Instead of a vista, I was head down, trying not to be completely pummelled. And instead of rejoicing and snapping pics at the summit, by the time I got there, I was photoless, hungry, and very cold.

That Day One trek ended about an hour later, after a sharp descent along the highway into Roncesvalles, at the historic pilgrim hostel. I'd walked nearly forty thousand steps in roughly ten hours and was exhausted. And if I hadn't booked a bed ahead of time, which thankfully I thought to do, I would have been out of luck. When I arrived, I heard them turning away people without reservations.

EXPECTING THE UNEXPECTED

I tell you this story as a cautionary tale for two reasons: First, if you are doing the Camino Francés from Saint-Jean-Pied-de-Port, the first day will be one of the most challenging of your trip. Especially if you decide to walk the entire distance between Saint-Jean-Pied-de-Port and Roncesvalles, on *either* the Napoleon or the Valcarlos routes through the Pyrenees. If you are nervous about this kind of first day being too much for you, I would highly recommend booking halfway accommodation. You may need to do this months in advance, as there aren't many options.

Second, I hope my experience shows how important it is to be able to roll with the punches. Your Camino will delight you, but it will also surprise you. Expect the unexpected!

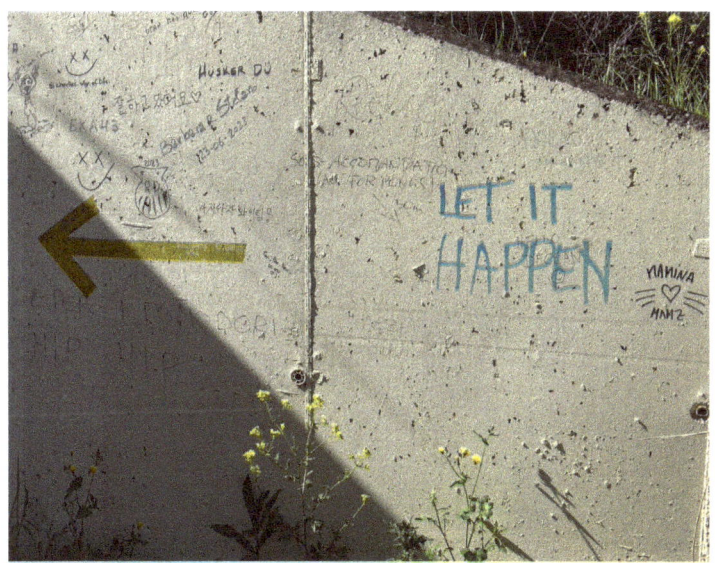

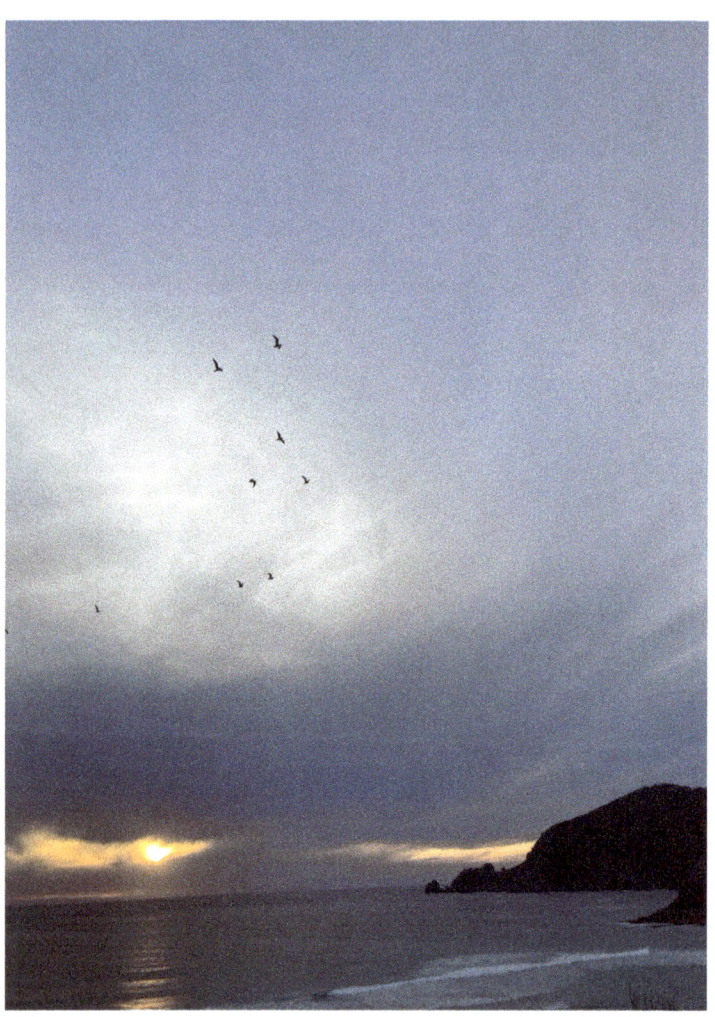

LISTENING TO YOUR BODY

On the morning of my third day, I had only walked about five kilometres before I had to stop on the side of the trail to rest and rub an aching knee. The back to back of a vigorous uphill on day one, followed by an extremely steep and treacherous downhill on day two, had taken a toll.

I had found a walking stick the day before to help take some of the strain off my knees and was already thinking I would need to buy poles in Pamplona, the first large city on the route.

Just at that moment, a French couple, who looked like they routinely hiked the Alps, stopped to check on me. This is one of the loveliest things about the Camino, and something I hadn't expected. Whenever you stop to rest, you can be guaranteed that someone will make sure you are doing okay, even if you have only stopped to have a small break and drink some water.

The French couple, who had no English, gestured to their sticks and their knees, nodding vigorously. With their sign language and my little bit of French, I could tell they were saying something like: "Why in the world are you walking without poles?!"

I smiled and nodded but felt embarrassed. How could I not have known I would need poles? Why hadn't I trained harder and better? Why did I have to rest when everyone else seemed fine?

For this Camino to truly be your own, you are going to have to learn to listen to your unique and individual body, respect what it needs, and be kind to yourself in the process. We all come to the Camino in different shapes, sizes, and states of fitness. We all have different injuries and weak spots. And it's of absolutely no use to compare yourself to others.

This might be difficult if you see pilgrims streaming past you. You may be tempted to be hard on yourself. "Why can't I walk any faster? Why am I struggling? What's wrong with me?" That inner critical voice can be hard to shake, but it's essential that you pay attention to what your body is telling you.

Do you need to stop and rest? Do you need to have a snack or water? Do you need to stretch? These are important questions to ask as you are walking, especially in the first few days, while your body is getting used to trekking such long distances, day after day.

There is no need to move more quickly than feels comfortable and no need to push through pain and angst when you can simply stop. Providing what your body is asking for is a crucial part of creating a journey that is both enjoyable and successful.

Anyone who has already walked the Camino can tell you stories of people they met who had to end their journey and fly home, often due to an injury. Your whole trip may be at risk if you don't tune into what you need or if you ignore the cues your body is sending. Please pay attention!

LISTENING TO YOUR BODY

As I mentioned earlier, many pilgrims have elaborate routines for taking care of their feet once blisters appear—body glide cream, Band-Aids, taping—but what about the whole body? Consider establishing a routine for how you are going to take care of yours.

A FEW BODY CARE TIPS:

- Consider a little bit of stretching for your feet, ankles, calves, hips, back, and shoulders at the beginning and end of each day. I took along a lightweight stretching band, which was excellent for loosening sore shoulders and hamstrings.

- Don't feel shy about taking breaks. Even ten minutes with your shoes and socks off while having a snack can make a big difference. There are so many beautiful places to stop—resting gives you time to enjoy the view!

- After each day's walk, find a spot where you can lie down and put your legs up a wall. Your bum should be tucked into the wall and your legs at a right angle to the floor. This elevation of the feet and legs helped me with both pain and swelling. I did this exercise faithfully, and on the one day I forgot, I definitely noticed how much this practice was helping!

- If you are someone who is used to a daily yoga or stretching routine, take advantage of albergues or hostels with outdoor green space and stretch your whole body in the soft grass. These opportunities are rare, and more often than not, you'll have to do modified stretches or poses in somewhat cramped spaces.

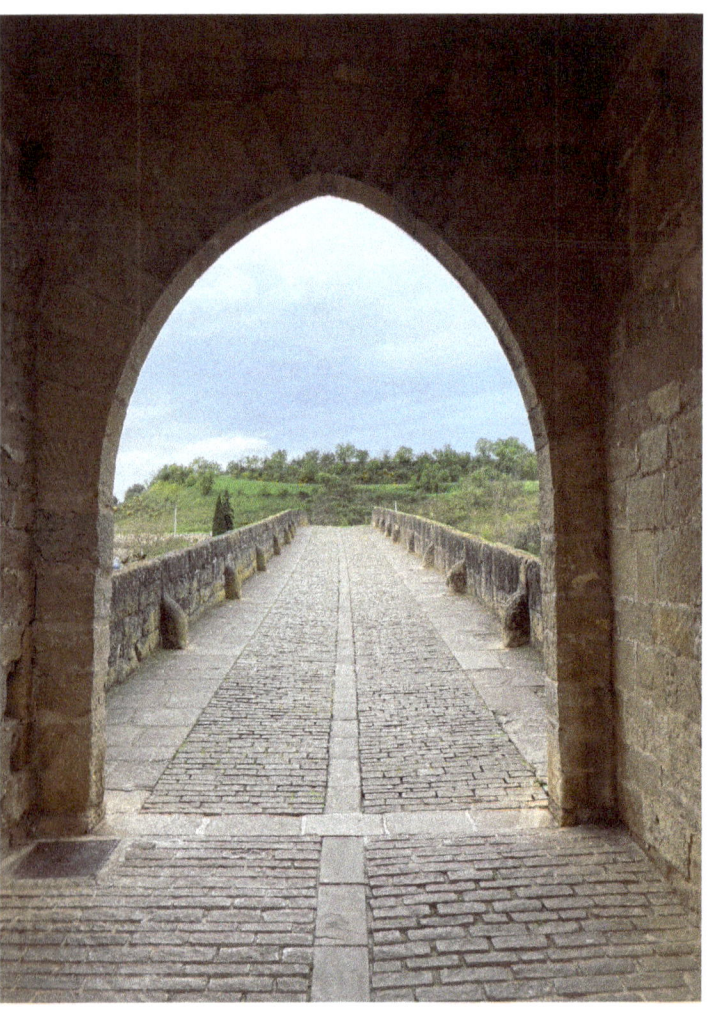

RESPECTING YOUR OWN NATURE

By the time I reached the first large city, Pamplona, I'd already made a decision that I didn't see coming: I booked a private room. Back at home, during my winter months of intense planning and budgeting, I gave myself permission to splurge on a private room a few times on the route. I imagined this would happen much later, a few weeks in, when I needed a little pampering.

That's how I thought of the need for a private room before I got to Spain: pampering. A hot shower without a lineup. And a bed with sheets. I inconveniently forgot that I am a real introvert and that being around people all the time would begin to exhaust me.

Once I got to Spain and began walking, a private room didn't just feel like pampering. It felt like a necessary expense for my introverted self. Just as my body was trying to acclimatize to carrying weight while traversing challenging terrain, so too was my spirit trying to get used to having people around all the time!

That's why I nearly dropped to my knees in gratitude when I entered the private room in Pamplona. I was so hungry for a space that was just my own.

If you are an introvert, the Camino may feel overwhelming at times. For those who don't know: an introvert is someone who recharges their batteries by being alone. Extroverts recharge their batteries by being with others. We introverts can get a bad rap and are often misunderstood. Some call us anti-social, shy, or boring, and don't understand why we might need space to quietly be by ourselves.

In some ways, the Camino is built for extroverts. You are surrounded by people— common sleeping quarters, a shared walking path, communal meals. If you're an introvert, you will need to work a little harder to ensure you get the time you need alone.

This was one of those things that I skimmed over in my preparation. I knew before the trip that I would need more space than most people and that I don't sleep well in a room full of others. But I had convinced myself that staying in albergues is what a "good pilgrim" should do (there are those Camino Rules again!). And anyway, I thought I'd be so tired it wouldn't matter. It did.

After Pamplona and for the rest of the Camino, I worked hard to respect the needs of my introverted self by booking solo rooms when I needed them. And in order to connect with others, I stayed open and receptive to conversations with other pilgrims and often sought out albergues with communal dinners, as I found this was a great way to get to know the strangers I would be sleeping in the same room with that night!

Give some thought to your own nature and what you will need on the Camino, and then plan ahead. If you know you are an extrovert and thrive on interactions with others, sleeping in albergues and perhaps even finding a "Camino family" whom you walk with every day might sound like bliss. And if you know you need a lot of introverted alone time, respect that, and seek out your solitude.

HONOURING CONNECTIONS

When I woke up in Pamplona, I knew I wanted to stay another day. I had spent the evening before visiting the outfitter shop and buying walking poles, scouting for supper, and shopping for snacks. There wasn't much time to really see the city. But I was keen to explore more of this beautiful place where Ernest Hemingway had spent so much time. I also felt that it would do my knees good to rest another day before hoisting my pack again.

The only hitch was that my first Camino friend, Elisa, whom I'd met on the train into Saint Jean, had already texted to say she was leaving Pamplona that morning. Over the previous few days, we'd crossed paths a few times, and I'd really enjoyed our conversations. She was two decades younger, though, and was used to carrying heavier packs for longer distances in the wilds of Arizona.

All that to say that in Pamplona, where I longed for a break, she was still raring to go. It was a bittersweet moment; I knew if we parted ways now, I would never catch up to her. And while I understood the importance of listening to my body and doing something for myself, it came at the cost of a lovely and blossoming friendship.

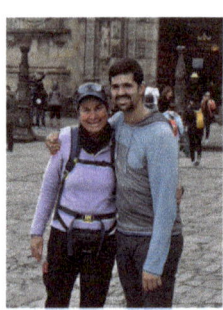
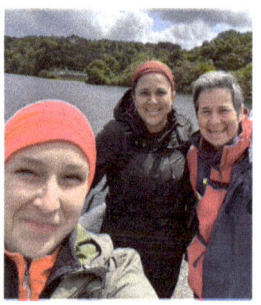
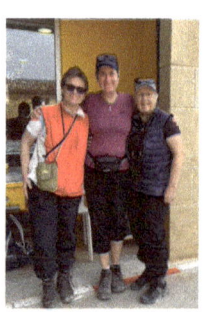
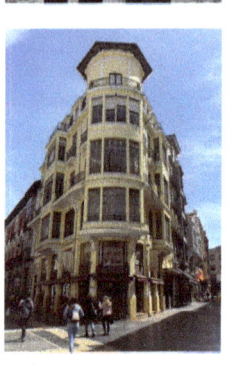
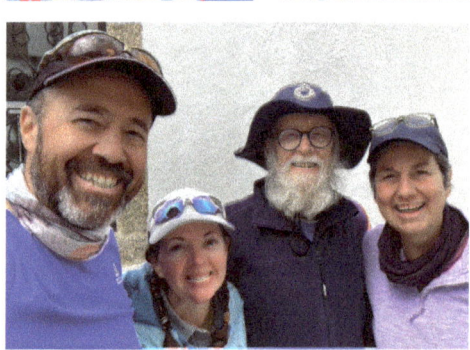
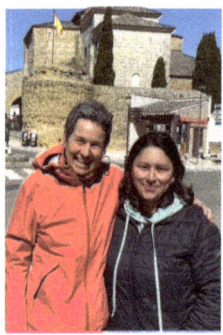
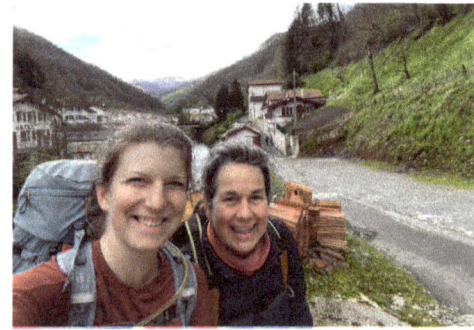

HONOURING CONNECTIONS

One of the very best parts of my Camino were the people I met along the way and the conversations we had that were both deep and meaningful. As I walked, I ended up talking to scores of people every day, some for only a few moments and others for hours.

These conversations all had a particular magic to them, something that I recalled from a backpacking trip I took in my twenties. An in-the-moment immediacy. An honest, soul-baring authenticity. An "I've got nothing to hide and nothing to lose" vulnerability.

It's a beautiful thing, and if you're open to it, these types of intimate connections can become a mainstay of your walk. I believe they are made possible by the reality of the situation you find yourself in—meeting people essentially by chance and not knowing how long your conversation or connection will last.

I thought often of the David Gray song *Say Hello, Wave Goodbye*, because on the Camino path, sometimes the moment of greeting was so quickly followed by the moment of farewell. You might meet someone very special and have a wonderful conversation, and then that person is gone, possibly never to be seen again!

I met some incredible people in the first few days of my trip whom I would have loved to see again, but that didn't happen. My advice to you is to take lots of photos of special people, and also remember to exchange contact information.

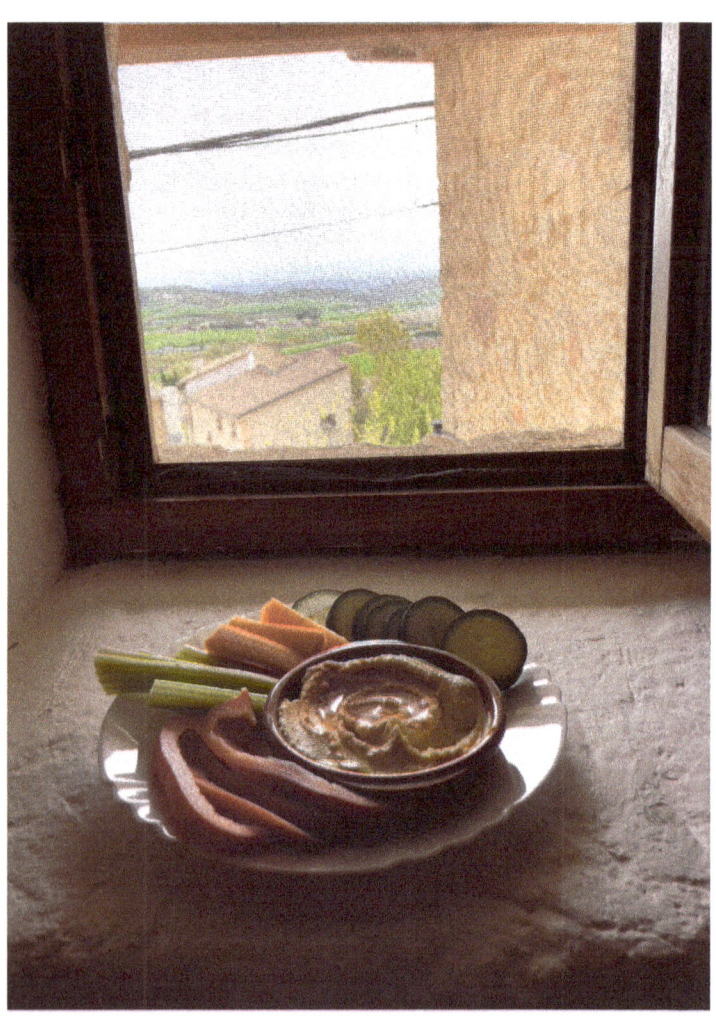

FEEDING YOURSELF

A few months before I walked the Camino, and after years of trying to figure out why I seemed to get every cold and flu that came along, I visited a naturopath who did a test that indicated I was intolerant to sugar and potatoes.

Over the years, this undiagnosed intolerance had led to a suppressed and less resilient immune system. And while I was happy to finally know this, my big trip was on the horizon, and I was worried about needing to avoid certain foods, especially in a foreign country.

In consultations with my Spanish teacher and also the Internet, I learned that there are definitely a lot of potatoes and sugar offered to pilgrims on the Camino! There is the ubiquitous tortilla (a Spanish omelette with potatoes, cut like a piece of pie) and churros (fried dough dipped in sugar and coated in chocolate), just to name two. So yes, I did miss out on some delicious treats (enjoy them if you're able!), but there was enough variety that I was able to find lots of other things to eat.

If you have existing food sensitivities, allergies, or intolerances, you are probably used to dealing with it. The added challenge when you walk the Camino will be doing this in another language! Before I left home, I memorized certain Spanish phrases and questions that enabled me to inquire about ingredients within meals along the way. This really helped.

Heads-up: Even if you're someone who can eat anything, finding food you like and that will sustain you can still be somewhat tricky on the Camino. It's a unique situation, after all. You are constantly on the move and can never be sure what will be on offer in the next town you reach.

That said, when you walk into a café in the morning at any point along the Camino, you can be assured that you will be able to get coffee, tea, and pastries. Often there is the tortilla I mentioned above, which is truly a Spanish staple. And if there is a kitchen, you can usually order an easy omelette (what Spaniards call Tortilla Francesca) or an "American-style" eggs and bacon, although ham (*jamón*) is more popular in Spain.

For lunch and supper, most restaurants (and some albergues and hostels) offer the pilgrim meal I mentioned earlier. You might get sick of eating the same thing and will want to seek out something else. I found myself desperately craving vegetables, which is why I hunted for albergues that boasted homemade meals.

The other option is to look for accommodation with kitchen access (your guidebook or apps can help with this). If you're someone who enjoys cooking and misses it, or you are craving variety or comfort food, finding a kitchen might really make your day. Grocery stores, especially the larger ones in bigger cities, are well stocked with items that will help you make a quick and healthy meal (bread, crackers, pastas, yoghurts, fruits, cheeses, etc.), plus your own coffee or tea in the morning before you head out! These kitchens often have leftover things in the fridge from the people who just left, so you might not even have to buy staples like milk or bread.

FEEDING YOURSELF

Here are a few additional tips about food from my experience:

- Cafés and restaurants might be closed when you pass by (many open in late morning and also close for a long siesta break in the afternoon), so having your own food supply is essential.

- I always walked with my own snacks, usually bananas, mandarins, and apples, plus granola bars, crackers, and cans of tuna. I would often have a snacky lunch rather than choosing a café or restaurant. This was more economical, plus I enjoyed eating my lunch outside under the shade of a tree or on a riverbank.

- It's important to remember that Spaniards eat their evening meal very late, mostly after eight p.m. You may luck into a restaurant or an albergue where you can get food by seven thirty, but usually not any earlier than that. If this feels too late for you, you may want to consider having a larger lunch and a light "snack supper" you prepare yourself.

- I am particular about my tea (maybe you are too?), so I brought my own tea bags from home. When I was staying somewhere with a communal kitchen facility, it was so nice to be able to make myself a cup of tea before I left in the morning.

One last thing to say about food: I'm not sure if everyone has this experience, but in the first ten days or so, due to the increased energy expenditure, I felt like I was always hungry. So, stocking up on snacks was essential!

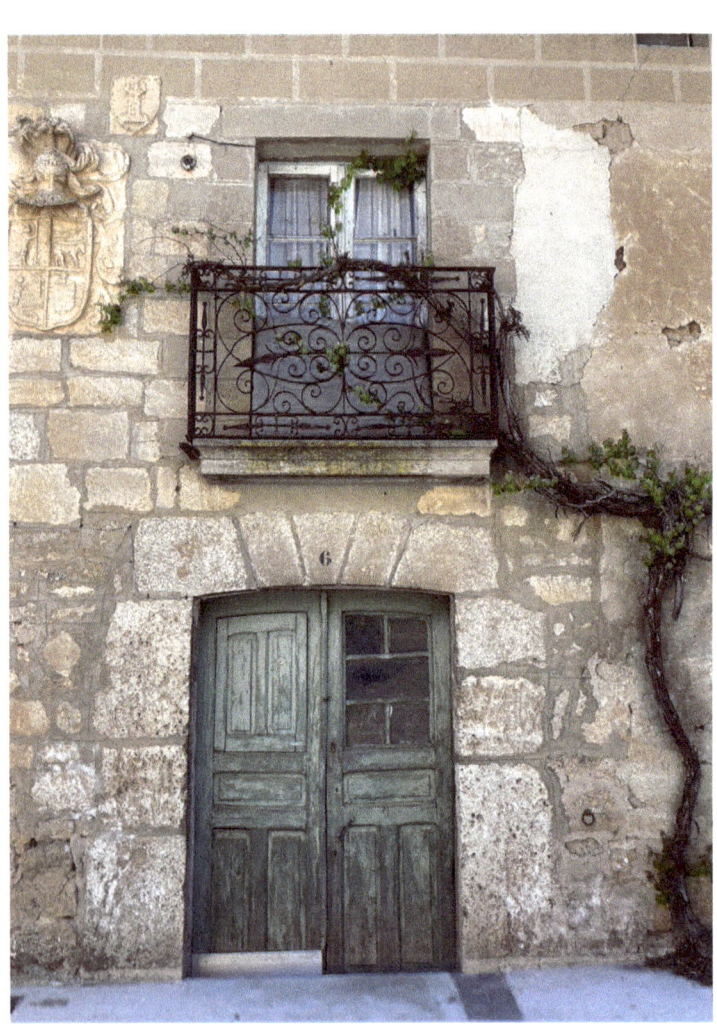

GOING OFF-STAGE

It was a beautiful day and I was sitting outside a clean, non-crowded albergue talking to the owner, a woman named Miren. She had set up a drying rack in the fresh air for my laundry, and we were in the middle of a deep conversation. We had cups of tea in our hands, suppertime was still hours away, and because there was only one other person in the dorm, Miren was not run off her feet and actually had time to sit with me.

I had noticed her tattoo, an elegant script with the Spanish word *confía*. She explained that *confía* means *trust* and that over the last few years, life had thrown her some unexpected curve balls. She had needed to learn to trust herself and to trust life as she navigated the challenges, and she'd gotten the tattoo as a reminder. As she spoke, I felt goosebumps erupt on my skin. Given my reason for walking the Camino—to learn to trust myself—this conversation felt like a synchronistic gift from the universe.

This moment in time remains one of the highlights of my Camino. Not only was it a chance meeting with a kindred spirit, but the sense of spaciousness I felt was directly related to a choice I had made two days earlier, as I left Pamplona. I had decided to go "off-stage."

If you've done any amount of research via websites or books about the Camino, you've likely run into the word *stages*. The

Camino Francés is usually divided into thirty-three stages of twenty to thirty kilometres each. These stages, each of which represents a day, include a starting point and an ending point and are configured so that if you follow the itinerary, you can do the Camino Francés in just over a month.

There are many people who walk according to the stages outlined in their guidebook and do not veer off the recommended distances or destinations. This leads to congestion! Pilgrims jockey for beds and food at the end points of each of the Camino stages, which tend to be the larger towns or cities.

When you decide to go off-stage, it means you are choosing to veer from the outlined stages by avoiding the traditional end points. For instance, on Day Four, leaving Pamplona, the guidebooks recommend Puente la Reina as that day's destination. Instead of ending there, I decided to find accommodation in the much smaller Obanos, about 2.5 km shy of Puente la Reina. I stayed in a house-turned-hostel on a quiet street, had a lovely supper with only one other pilgrim, and then a fabulous sleep.

On Day Five, I did the same thing, stopping 4 km from the recommended endpoint of Estella and lucking into the gift of Miren and her wonderful albergue in Villatuerta.

Once I decided to go off-stage, I felt like I'd discovered a real secret in terms of avoiding crowds. This way of walking might not be for everyone, but if you are someone who doesn't like following the pack and craves more independence, quiet, and solitude, I highly recommend it.

GOING OFF-STAGE

On the Camino Francés, there is a built-up infrastructure all along the path, not just in the larger cities and towns. This means that even in smaller towns and villages there is always somewhere to stay. The added bonus of going off-stage is that sometimes the accommodation is a little bit less expensive!

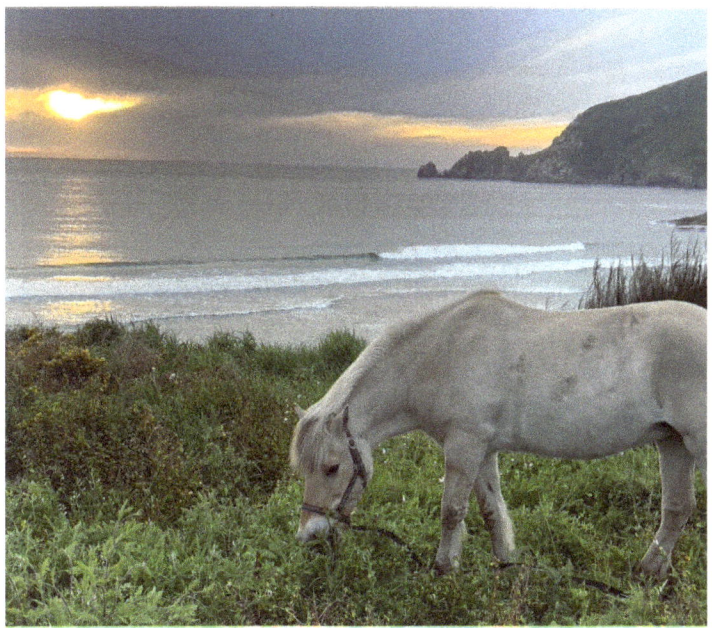

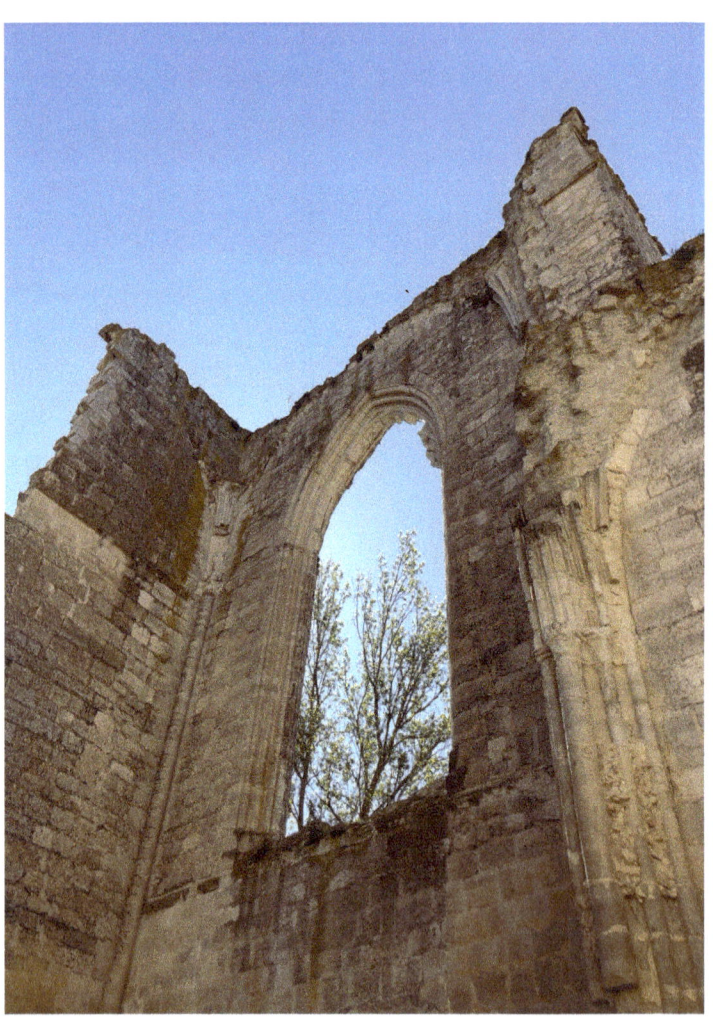

KEEPING YOUR EYES UP

The birds were singing, the path through the fields was lined with beautiful spring flowers, and to my delight, within a couple of kilometres of leaving the previous night's accommodation, I came across a ruin.

When I checked my guidebook, I discovered it was Ermita de San Miguel, an ancient pilgrim hospital and a tenth-century hermitage. Over one thousand years old! Coming from Canada, where the oldest buildings are about 250 years old, this felt very special indeed.

The ruin was only a little ways off the Camino trail, so I decided to stop. There was no one else around, and when I stepped through the doorway, I felt a cool, calm stillness. As my eyes adjusted, I could see a stone altar along the wall, covered in paper and objects. I approached and took in what can only be described as a glorious and eclectic offering: rocks, shells, feathers, photos, a bracelet, a glass jar with dried flowers, and reams of handwritten papers, torn from notebooks.

There were prayers for others ("Please help heal Nonna and return her to health."), gratitude for the journey ("San Miguel, saints and angels, whoever hears: thank you, thank you, thank you."), and heartfelt pleas ("My heart feels so heavy. I am so lonely, even here.

Please be with those who are lonelier than I and show me where the world is bigger than me. Show me how to understand.").

These notes made my eyes well up with tears as I imagined other pilgrims standing in this sacred space, writing these notes to something larger than themselves, daring to hope for healing or freedom from what troubled them.

Quiet, contemplative moments like this were the heart of my Camino. In retrospect, it seems now that the more I planned, the more my plans went awry. And the more I went with the flow and appreciated what was being offered to me, the richer my journey became.

I want to encourage you to make plans if they make you feel comfortable but not to do so much research and forward planning that you miss out on surprises like this one. I saw a lot of walkers who marched right past places like this because they were hell-bent on getting to their destination.

Even if you have every day mapped out to the last kilometre, remember to keep your eyes up when you're on the path. You'd be surprised how many pilgrims I saw looking down at their feet as they walked. Making sure you don't trip and fall is important but so is being open and receptive to the history and the stories of the country you're in.

The Camino is filled with these types of ancient relics, with only small signs indicating they are even there. Stay attentive, be curious, and allow yourself time to stop and take in some of these hidden gems.

TAKING CARE OF BUSINESS

You may have already secretly googled "Where do I go to the bathroom on the Camino?" If you feel shy or nervous about this topic, you're in the right place. If, however, you are already a pro outdoor eliminator, used to hiking and camping and having to answer the call of nature outside, go ahead and skip this chapter.

When you walk the Camino, you are likely going to have to pee, and maybe poop, outside. I'm sorry if this comes as a surprise, but the best thing you can do is prepare yourself!

There are vast stretches in between towns with no toilet facilities in sight, but even if you are walking through a town, there is no guarantee you will be able to find an open establishment with a toilet. There are very few public washrooms in Spain, and if you happen to be passing through a town at siesta time, restaurants and cafés—the places that are likely to have toilets—will not be open. FYI: Siesta time can stretch anywhere between one and five p.m.!

And it's not just afternoons that can be tricky for finding bathroom facilities. Early in the morning can also be dicey! There were times when I left early and passed through two or three places that were like ghost towns, all shuttered up. No place to pee for ten kilometres or more!

Many women pilgrims are prepared, with toilet paper or tissue for these situations, but sadly, many also leave them behind! Please do NOT do this! I can't tell you how many paper tissues or pieces of toilet paper I saw lying on the ground along the Camino. People who would never throw a bottle or a can out of a car window on the highway and who "reduce, reuse, recycle" at home don't even seem to think twice about leaving tissue or toilet paper on the path. Yes, they will decompose eventually, but it takes a very long time for that to happen, and in the meantime, what is left is an eyesore for everyone who passes by.

Here are a few options for you to consider in your pee and poop preparation!

- Carry a plastic bag for your pee tissues and then dispose of them in the next town.

- Better yet, use a piece of cloth that you already have, like a bandana, and wash it out when you do your daily laundry.

- If that idea grosses you out, consider a reusable, antimicrobial "pee cloth" (available at most outfitter shops). Some of these even have a snap function so that once it is used, it can be snapped onto the outside of your backpack to dry in the sun. Added bonus: They are bacteria- and odour-resistant!

- Consider buying a "female urination device" (of which there are many!) that enables you to pee standing up. If you've never heard of this, just google the term above and you'll be amazed. Pro tip: Practise at home before you pack it to make sure you understand how it works!

TAKING CARE OF BUSINESS

- When it comes to pooping, the best thing for everyone, and for all of nature, is to not do this outside. But if it's an emergency, make sure to go far off the trail and dig what is called a "cat hole." Some people even carry a special lightweight "poop trowel" (available online). Poop in the hole, cover it up, and carry your toilet paper out.

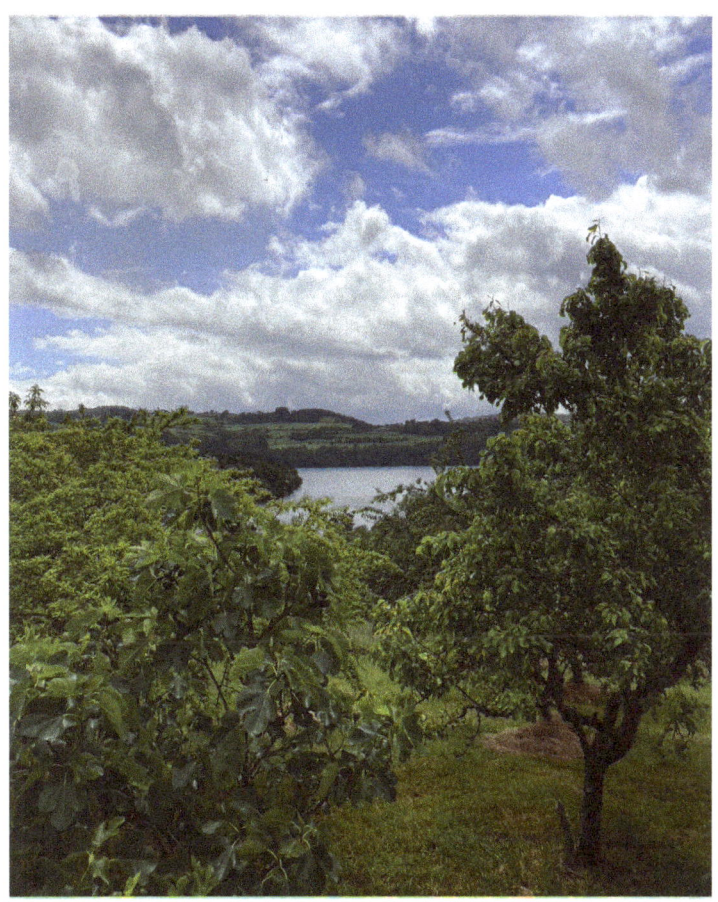

THE MIDDLE

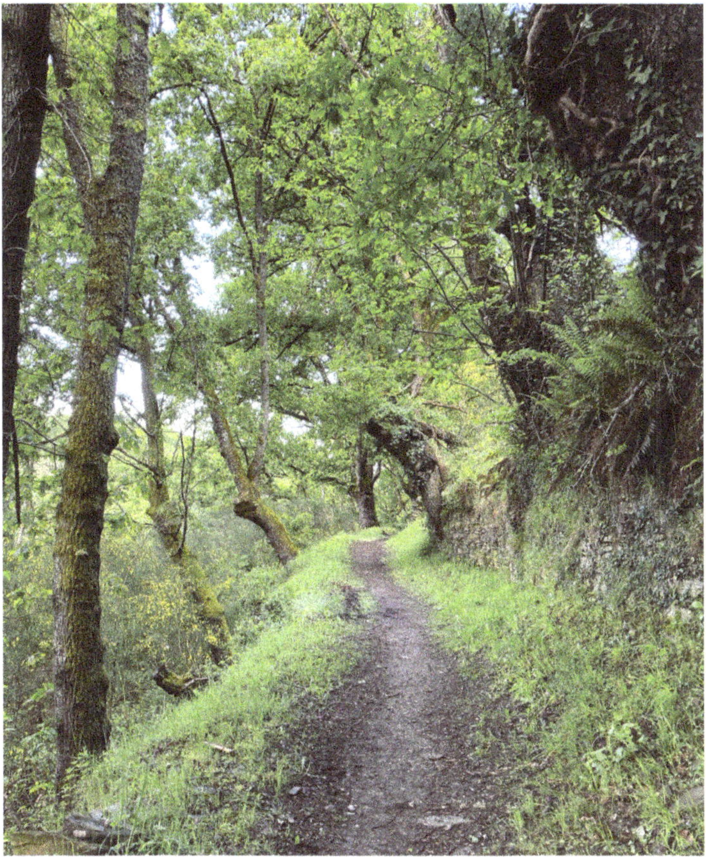

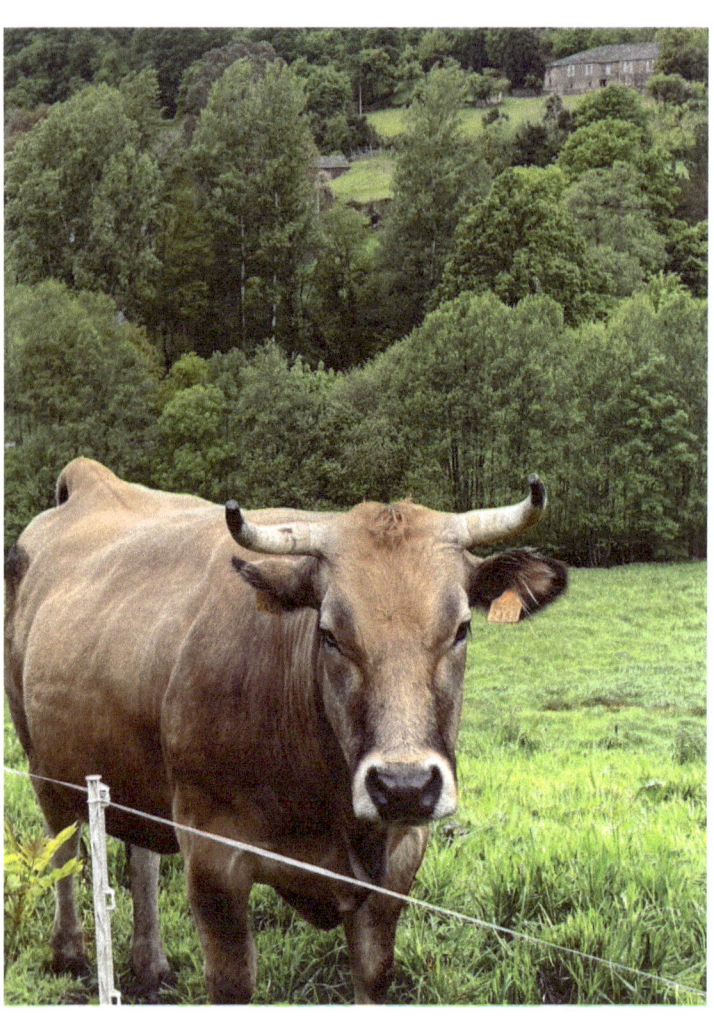

FINDING HUMOUR

I couldn't get out of there fast enough.

The reviews for this albergue run by a religious community had been all positive. One of the reviews had even said: "Don't worry. They won't push their religion on you."

Ha! At supper I was seated with people I thought were other pilgrims, but they turned out to be volunteers with the religious community. I was the only Camino walker at our table. And rather than having ordinary conversation—Where are you from? How long have you been here? How do you like Spain?—I was peppered with intrusive questions from all five sides. Actually, peppered is the wrong word; it felt more like machine-gun fire. I could barely eat my supper!

They stared at me earnestly, asking question after question about my religious orientation and my spiritual life and my reasons for walking the Camino. I casually inserted that my partner was a woman and that we had a blended family with three children, hoping they would turn away in disgust because I was living in sin. But that's when they switched tactics and launched into "testimony" about how they had found Jesus and how much better their life had been since then. Sigh. There was no doubt they were trying to "save my soul." Deeply uncomfortable, I feigned a sore stomach and went to bed early.

In the morning, I left while it was still dark, creeping down the stairs with a flashlight, only to find the main door bolted and locked. I told myself funny stories about how they trap and convert pilgrims while I fiddled with the mechanics of the door, finally figuring it out. Hallelujah! The still dark, cool morning smelled delicious with freedom as I found the yellow arrows that mark the Camino path and was on my way.

I want to assure you that I am not anti-religion. This community felt more like a cult. I also want to assure you that this kind of experience is a very uncommon one, although there are all kinds of discomforts you may experience along the way.

Whether you're wide awake in the middle of the night with a room full of snorers, or you witness something disturbing or unsettling, there will undoubtedly be some strained moments. This is what happens when you spend time walking, eating, and sleeping in close proximity to others, all from a variety of different backgrounds.

Don't worry! As my Scottish great-grandmother used to say, "This too shall pass." Trying to find the humour in challenging situations also really helps.

And so does the light of day! Every time I had a rough night, I was always soooo happy to push open the door onto a fresh start the next morning. Remember, happiness isn't the absence of problems, strange encounters, or difficult situations. It's what we do with these challenging experiences that make all the difference.

ENJOYING THE MORNINGS

The morning of my escape from the cultish albergue was the earliest I got up and hit the path. And I'm so glad I did. The sunrise was gorgeous, and it inspired me to set my alarm a little bit earlier on subsequent days. These are some of my favourite memories of the Camino: the first five or six kilometres of any given day, just as the sky was lightening, bird song filling the air around me.

At home, early mornings are usually dedicated tea drinking and writing time, but on the Camino, they became a time to quietly pack and start walking. I often felt that I had the Camino path all to myself, with the added bonus of getting to the next night's stay a little earlier in the day.

If you are a morning person already—and even if you aren't—I highly recommend getting an early start when you're walking. In addition to the beauty and the quiet, it's also much cooler if you are battling heat!

Tip: If you are a bird lover, download the Cornell Lab Merlin app for the region you'll be in before you leave home. It was so fun to stop and let the app listen in an area where there was a lot of birdsong. It identifies the birds via their song and generates an in-the-moment list of all the birds around you.

The Eurasian blackcap, nuthatch, and robin; the European serin, goldfinch, and greenfinch; the corn bunting, the Cetti's warbler, and the Eurasian scops owl. Plus the cuckoo, the nightingale, and the crested lark. This is a short list of just *some* of the birds I heard.

It was fascinating and a way for me to feel like I was learning as I was walking.

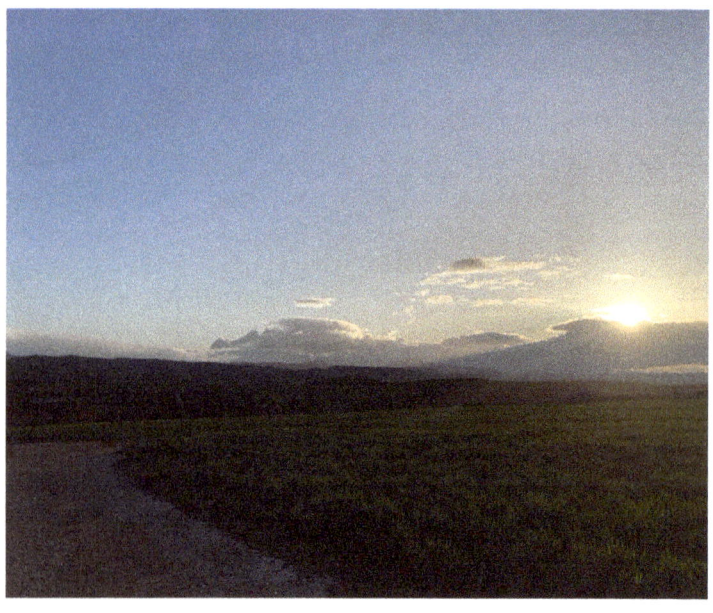

CHOOSING WATER OVER WINE

Have you ever heard of the Irache wine fountain on the Camino Francés? Back when I used to drink, the idea of a fountain of wine sounded exotic and enticing. But on the day when I found myself approaching it, after almost eight years without a drink, I didn't feel excited. I felt nervous.

There were enormous signs about the upcoming wine fountain, and as I saw each one, I imagined the place crowded with pilgrims. I envisioned the gathered group calling to me and inviting me in. How would I say no without feeling stodgy and no fun?

The drinking culture of the Camino was something I'd been worried about as I planned my trip. It stood in contrast to my home social life where I mostly hang out with people who don't drink or drink very little.

"No vino, no Camino." That was a T-shirt I'd seen on Day Two. Uh-oh, I thought. I'd already had to turn down wine on the first night at my hostel in Saint-Jean-Pied-de-Port, said no to the free wine on offer with the pilgrim's meal in Roncesvalles, and watched as others had a beer alongside their morning coffee. Yikes.

And now, here I was trudging up a dusty road toward the fountain, feeling lonely and longing for the accompaniment of my partner. If Malve had been with me, she would have reminded me that my decision not to drink was a good one. She would have told me I was strong. "You've got this," she would have said.

When I got to the wine fountain, I was surprised to find it sequestered behind a fence with not another soul around. It didn't look half as fun as I'd always imagined. It was just a modern-day tap set up on the outside wall of a local winery building. No crowds of boisterous pilgrims. No encouragement to break my commitment to myself. No massive fun-having that I felt on the outside of. I breathed a sigh of relief and kept walking.

If you are also a non-drinker, please don't let the fact that you don't drink stop you from walking the Camino. While it's true that there is a lot of drinking on offer, there is so much more available to you. Yes, you will see groups of people (usually very young men) stopping in every town to drink. And yes, you will be offered wine at pilgrim suppers and the like. But it is not the predominant vibe of the Camino, and you can easily choose not to be a part of it.

Here are a few insights and tips that I hope will help to ease your mind if you have worries that are similar to mine:

- There are A LOT of alcohol-free options available in the restaurants, bars, and cafés along the way: Zero Beer, Aquarius (a hydrating drink in a can), and Mosto (a delicious red or white grape juice).

- You will meet other people who also don't drink or drink very little. You won't be the only one! I was actually surprised at the number of pilgrims I encountered who were non-drinkers, and all for different reasons.

- Contrary to my imaginings about the zealous, pushy pilgrims at the wine fountain, no one I met on the path ever tried to talk me into having a drink! There was zero social pressure.

- If you can, be honest with the people you meet about the fact that you don't drink. Being truthful about something that is challenging or that we feel vulnerable about can help us stay the course. It also gives others permission to share more of their real selves with us too.

- If you are in the AA program, I have heard there are meetings in certain towns on the Camino. If this is part of your support strategy, I would recommend you look this up beforehand so you know which towns offer AA meetings and plan accordingly.

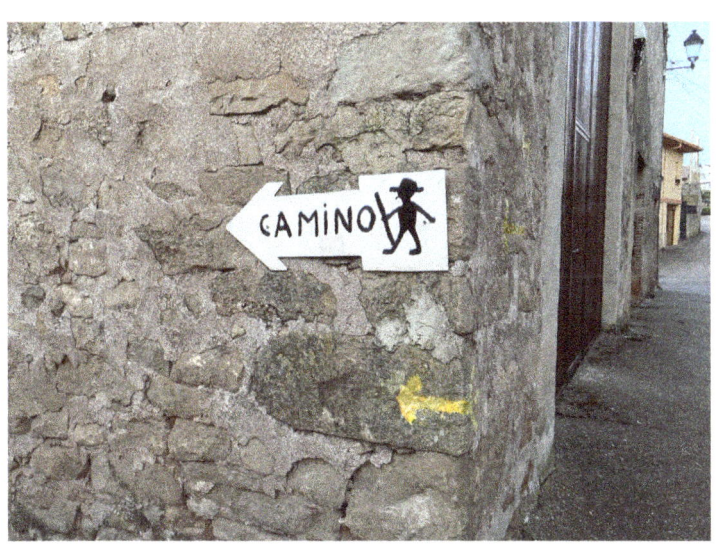

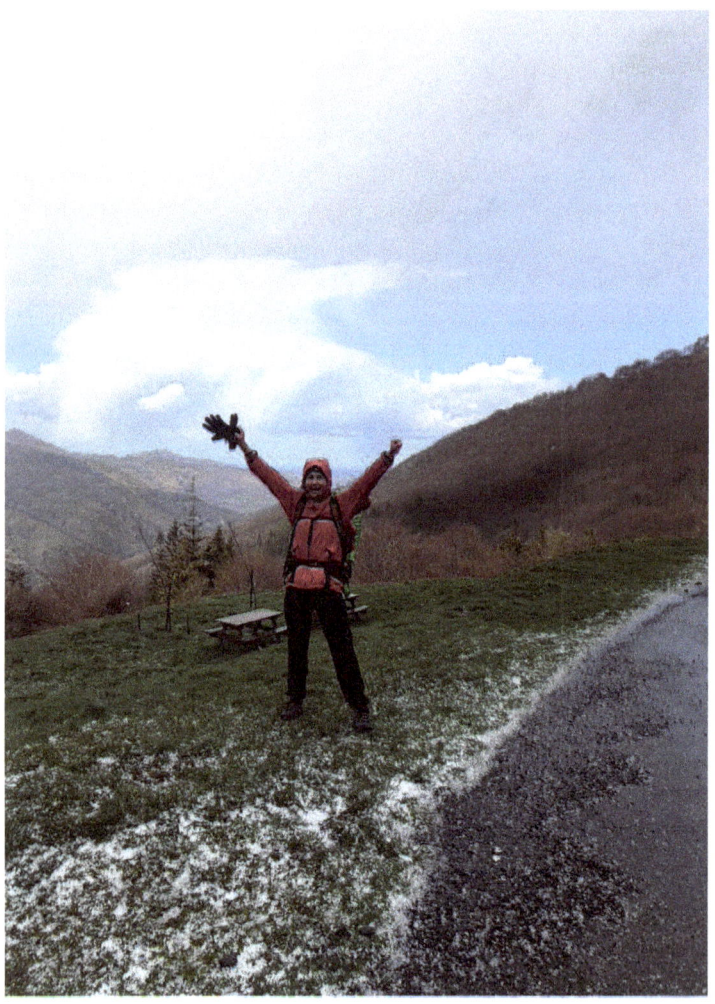

REACHING FOR JOY

I had just landed in a lovely albergue that had laundry facilities and a beautiful green space outside. I should have been elated and enjoying myself, but instead, I was on a video call with my partner and was crying my eyes out.

The night before, I had stayed in a crowded albergue where, in the middle of the night, someone in the small dorm room decided to call home and have a conversation in a normal talking voice. While everyone else was sleeping! He was talking so loudly that my earplugs didn't help at all and neither did a pillow over my head. It went on for at least an hour, and even after he hung up, I couldn't get back to sleep.

As soon as I saw the first light, I escaped from the dorm and went upstairs to the kitchen for breakfast. I ate, had my tea, and as soon as other people started waking up, I went back down to the dorm room, packed my stuff, and left.

The lack of sleep made for a difficult day. My body was tired, my feet were sore, my knee was swollen, and it was hot to boot. By the time I got to my destination, having walked the last few kilometres with no shade, I was depleted. All it took was seeing Malve's face on my phone screen and the tears started to flow. I berated myself for being a terrible pilgrim, for being whiny, and for not having fun when both of us had sacrificed so much to get me to Spain.

All to which she was super supportive and kind. "Go easy on yourself. You're doing a really big thing," she said. "Think of your Camino like having a baby. No matter how many books you've read or how many people you've talked to, you actually have no idea what it's like until it happens. And then suddenly you have a kid and you're like *oh shit*."

Was she ever right! Regardless of all the research I'd done, I had no idea what the Camino would actually be like until I was walking it. I think I had expected a feeling of near constant happiness and pride, despite physical pain that might surface. I wasn't expecting existential angst.

But existential angst was what I got. Fuelled by lack of sleep, I wondered what I was doing and why I thought this was a good idea. I felt lonely, in pain, and ragged from my exertions.

Malve said something else really important that day: "Don't lose the joy in the journey." This was the perfect piece of advice. She was right. I was supposed to be enjoying myself! And I had to figure out how to do that, even in the midst of lack of sleep, loneliness, and aches and pains.

After this little pep talk, I decided to intentionally plan relaxing, fun, and joyful things even if it made my day longer or meant I didn't walk as far. The very next day I made a point of stopping on a bench under an olive tree and actually lying down for a rest. The day after that, I took some time out to tour a cathedral and walk up a bell tower to take in the view. It was 134 steps up but well worth it!

REACHING FOR JOY

I want to note that adding activities or stops can be complicated. If you have a return ticket home and need to cover a certain number of kilometres each day, it might feel difficult to take time out. So, if you are pressed for time, try to remember to reach for the joy in the simple things: in each step, each conversation, each flower, each breeze, and every *café con leche* or delicious piece of tortilla.

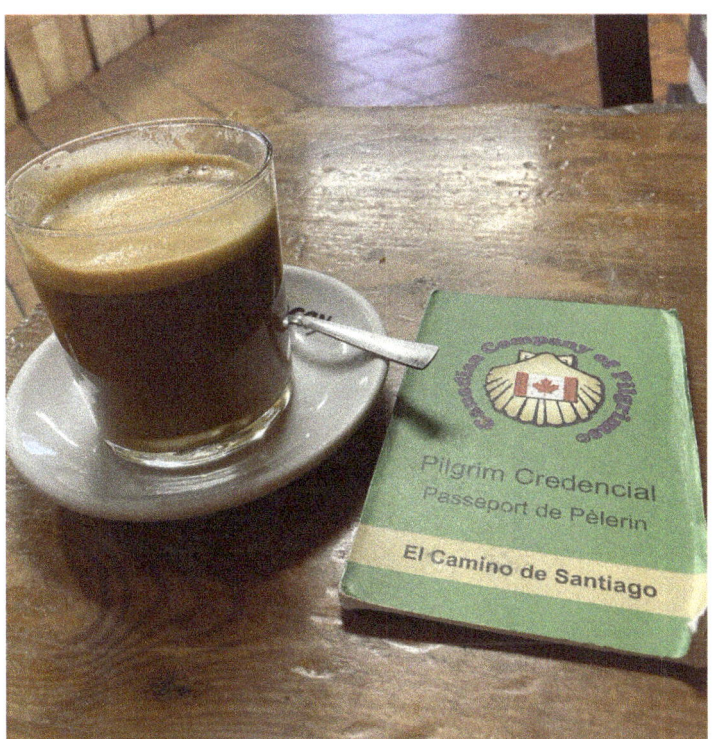

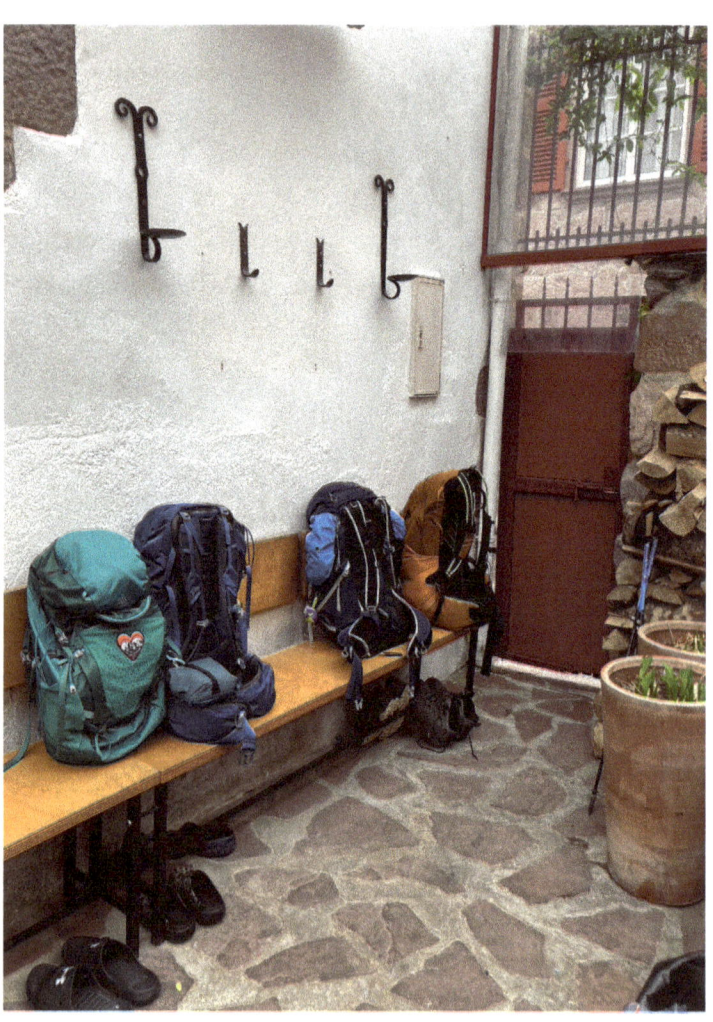

ALLOWING REST DAYS

Travelling alone and being independent is amazing in many ways, but you may sometimes feel lonely and suffer from decision fatigue.

When you walk the Camino solo, there are all kinds of decisions to make each and every day. Where to stay, where to eat, what to eat, who to talk to, how to tend to yourself, etc. Sometimes it gets a little tiring. On certain days, I remember wishing for someone to bounce things off of as I grappled with all the choices the Camino had to offer.

If any of this happens for you, it's possible you just need a rest day to regroup and re-energize. I highly recommend building days into your itinerary where you don't walk. You'll physically need them! Plus, there is an emotional bonus. Days that are devoted to simply "being," rather than moving onto the next place, are a real gift.

Keep those rest days in your pocket and use them when you really need them. You may choose a quiet place, somewhere to sit in a patch of sun and gaze at the trees and listen to the birds. Or you may be attracted to a bigger city.

Living in a city myself, I thought for sure that I would want to avoid the big cities and rest in smaller towns. I was wrong! While there is much to enjoy about the small towns on the Camino—ancient churches, cobblestone streets, cozy cafés, and the absolute quiet at siesta time—I revelled in the liveliness and bustle of the larger cities. And I loved how so much life goes on in the public squares. So different from North American culture!

It's very freeing to wake up on a rest day, knowing you don't have to walk and can stay where you are. First off, you don't need to pack up! And second, you have a chance to listen to your body and what it needs. Sightseeing? Taking a nap? Browsing in a bookstore? Whether you're sitting in one of the lively public squares, taking in a historic site, or simply wandering aimlessly, chances are that you are creating joyful moments and memories.

If you have the freedom to book a longer trip for yourself, I recommend taking as many rest days as you would like in the places that interest you. The Camino is more than just walking, and you want to make sure to get the most out of the country you have the good fortune to be passing through.

COPING WITH HEAT

I had just finished walking twenty-eight kilometres in a second day of blazing heat and had checked into a small family-run guesthouse. I'd had a shower, came down for supper, and joined a table of pilgrims.

It was while I was in the shower that I realized I had forgotten to put sunscreen on the backs of my legs. They were lobster-red. I sat beside a friend I'd met the day before, a lovely woman from Italy. I raised the back of my pants to show her the damage. "Mamma mia!" she gasped. It was pretty bad.

At that dinner, there were pilgrims from Germany, Italy, France, and the Netherlands. I was the only native English-speaker, but of course, as often happens on the Camino, everyone switched to the language we all had in common—no matter how halting—and I benefitted. I was very aware of my privilege every time I met people from other countries who continuously and graciously switched over to speak my mother tongue, not theirs.

We chatted about how our Caminos were going, shared photos of our families, and exchanged WhatsApp numbers so we could update each other on where we were. We also wondered aloud at how long the heat wave would continue and talked about how we'd all expected cooler temps in April.

What I didn't know then was that the blistering heat would continue for three more days, and I would wind up sick as a dog forty-two kilometres down the road (don't worry, that story is coming).

Depending on the route you take and what time of year you decide to walk the Camino, heat will likely be something you have to contend with.

Here are some tips for walking long distances in the Spanish heat (some of which I learned later but wish I had known about!):

- Consider walking a shorter distance on a day that you know is going to be extremely hot. If that is not possible, start your day early. If you begin walking at six or seven a.m., you will probably be at your destination by twelve or one p.m. Walking in scorching sunshine at two or three in the afternoon is no fun!

- Drink loads of water, and at least once or twice a day, add electrolyte tabs or packets when you fill your bottle.

- Every time you stop for water, splash cold water on your hands and face, and then soak a handkerchief or bandana and tie it around your neck. The cold drips feel delicious on your skin and will keep you cooler for longer.

- If it's a full sun day with very little opportunity for shade, make sure to stop in the shade you do come across. You don't know when the next shady spot will be!

COPING WITH HEAT

- A ball cap just won't cut it on days that are sweltering. Make sure you bring along a hat with a wide brim all the way around. I didn't have one of these and ended up buying one at an outfitter shop.

- A shade umbrella is also an option. I saw a few walkers with these, some with the miniature kind that is attached to a hat!

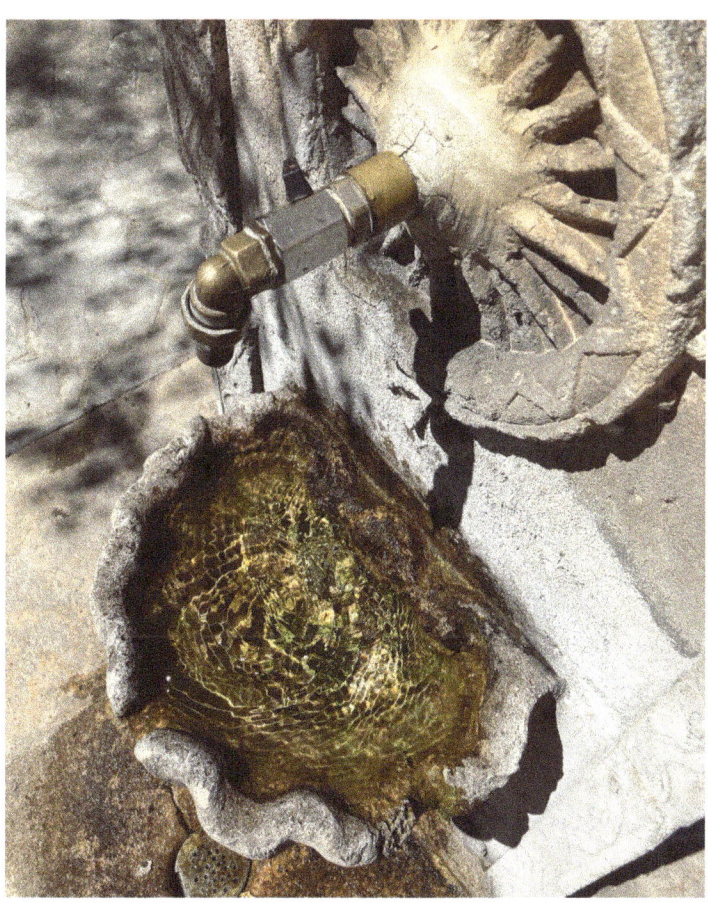

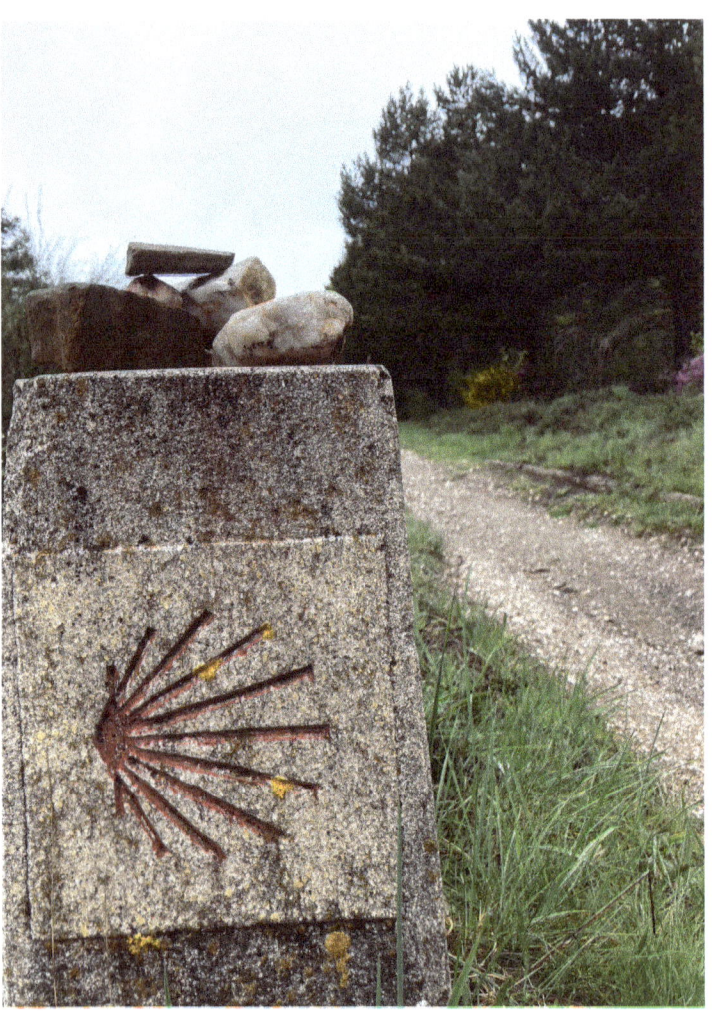

OVERCOMING CHALLENGES

The walking day had been long and incredibly hot, and there had been very little shade in between towns. Around the water fountains, pilgrims filled their bottles, dumped electrolytes in, and lamented about the heat and the fact that it was siesta time and there were no cool indoor places to rest.

I had created more shade for myself by draping a scarf underneath my ball cap and resting when I found shade, but even still, by the time I was trudging the last few kilometres of the day, I felt lightheaded and "off."

But it wasn't until after my shower that I started to feel very unwell. I had been planning on meeting a friend for supper at the restaurant next door, but instead I cancelled and, intuiting what was coming, headed to the store for hydrating drinks, instant oatmeal, and bland crackers. I made it back just in time for the onset of the vomiting and diarrhea that continued through the rest of the evening and into the night.

In between trips to the communal bathroom (awkward!), I wondered what was going on and considered whether or not I should be seeking help. Heat exhaustion? The breakfast I'd had at the roadside bar that morning? Maybe the flu?

By the time the sun came up, I was exhausted and depleted and knew there was no way I could walk that day. Burgos, one of the larger cities on the Camino, was only thirty kilometres away, and I figured if I was going to be sick, a bigger city might be a better place to be. Through my sickly haze, I managed to book a room in a hostel on my phone. I just needed to figure out how to get there.

The bus was the answer, although it was not the answer I wanted or had planned for. Like many other pilgrims, I had intended to walk all the way across Spain. I hadn't given a lot of thought to the notion that something might happen that would get in the way.

The kind owner of the albergue explained the bus system to me, made me a cup of ginger tea, and even walked me to the bus stop. I laid my head against the window and felt grateful that the Imodium I'd packed as an emergency medical supply seemed to be working. There was no toilet on the bus! Within thirty minutes I was in Burgos.

My illness, whatever it was (and I still don't know for sure!), lasted ten days. I wasn't in bed the whole time, but I was for the first three. After taking the bus into Burgos, I was stuck at a hostel without kitchen facilities, making peppermint tea and instant oatmeal with hot tap water. Not ideal!

Even though I knew I couldn't walk and that it was smart to take the bus and be closer to medical facilities, I was still heartbroken to miss walking part of the route. I had assumed because I was fit and healthy that I would be able to walk every step. It simply never occurred to me that I might become so sick I couldn't walk. It wasn't what I had expected or planned for, and I felt disappointed in this turn of events.

Things happen on the Camino—stuff you don't expect, stuff you can't even properly prepare for—and some of these things will challenge your most cherished ideas or hopes for your trip.

What I want to say to you is that even if you do experience a debilitating injury or an illness, it doesn't necessarily mean your Camino is over. It just means you may need to rethink your plan. If this happens, I want to encourage you to try and find the humour (if possible!) and also remember to be kind to yourself. This is the kind of trip where things can easily go awry and where you may need to alter your expectations and intentions.

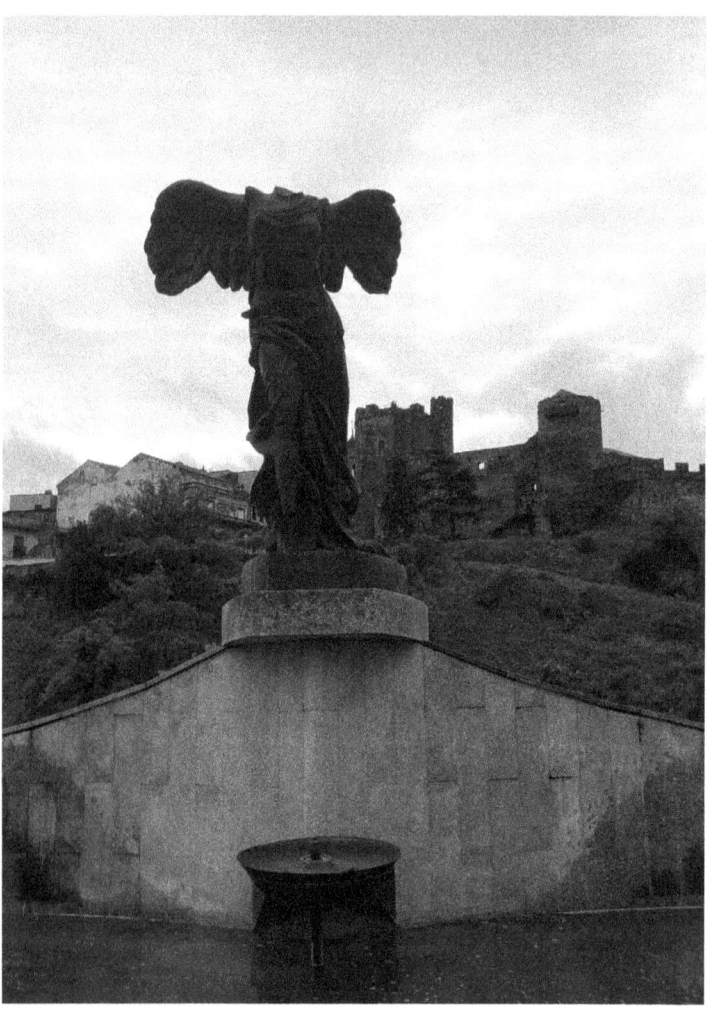

BATTLING THE INNER CRITIC

Being sick threw my whole itinerary off, and when I was finally able to walk again, I needed shorter days. I was also too weak from lack of food to carry my own bag and had to use a luggage transfer service. This was another of those unchecked assumptions I'd made before the trip began. Of course I would be carrying my bag the entire way! This is what I thought until I was faced with a situation I hadn't prepared for.

The first twenty-kilometre day I was attempting since getting sick just happened to coincide with the start of the Meseta, a plateau stretching between mountain ranges in the interior of Spain. The road stretched out before me, long and flat. After four days of a banana-and-oatmeal diet, I felt undernourished and deflated. To add insult to injury, I was still suffering from intermittent diarrhea, which made walking through areas without services nerve-wracking. Ugh.

And of course, that's when my inner critic knew to attack, just when my defences were down. When what I really needed was encouragement and support and maybe even kudos for continuing on, my critic started lobbing stink bombs at me instead.

You fail at everything you try. This walk is no exception. You had to take a bus, and now you're not even carrying your own bag. It's just embarrassing. This walk is an example of how completely and utterly selfish you are. Your partner is holding down the fort at home all by herself, and what are you doing? Walking. That's it. And you can't even do that right.

My critic always reserves its most cutting and vicious attacks for when I'm sick and have no ability to defend myself. This time was no exception—it was like I had completely forgotten how to be kind to myself. I wish on that day on the Meseta that I had been able to tell myself that getting sick was out of my control. I wish I'd been able to reach for compassion and understanding instead.

The compassionate message I needed arrived in a text later that night. It was from my American friends Kellie and Peter, whom I had met in Saint Jean. "So sorry to hear you've been sick. We're so impressed with your strength, when most of us would have given up and gone home. Your daughter will be so proud of you. And so are we!"

Those are the words I wish I could have been able to tell myself earlier that day. Tough, not wimpy. Strong, not weak. A survivor, not a failure. Take that, inner critic!

That text from my friends ignited a new approach to my challenges. Rather than being hard on myself, I began trying to embrace the "shit happens" (literally) mantra. There wasn't anything I could do about the fact that I had gotten sick and had "lost" time, but what I could control were my own thoughts and attitude about what lay ahead. As I started to feel physically stronger over the next few days, I set the intention to be kinder to myself.

There is a lot of time to think when you're walking for hours every day. And in choosing to walk the Camino alone, you create spaciousness in your mind for all kinds of thoughts to creep in, positive or negative. If you tend to be hard on yourself, this might be fertile ground for your inner demons to attack. Be prepared with a readiness to be kind and compassionate to yourself. No matter what happens.

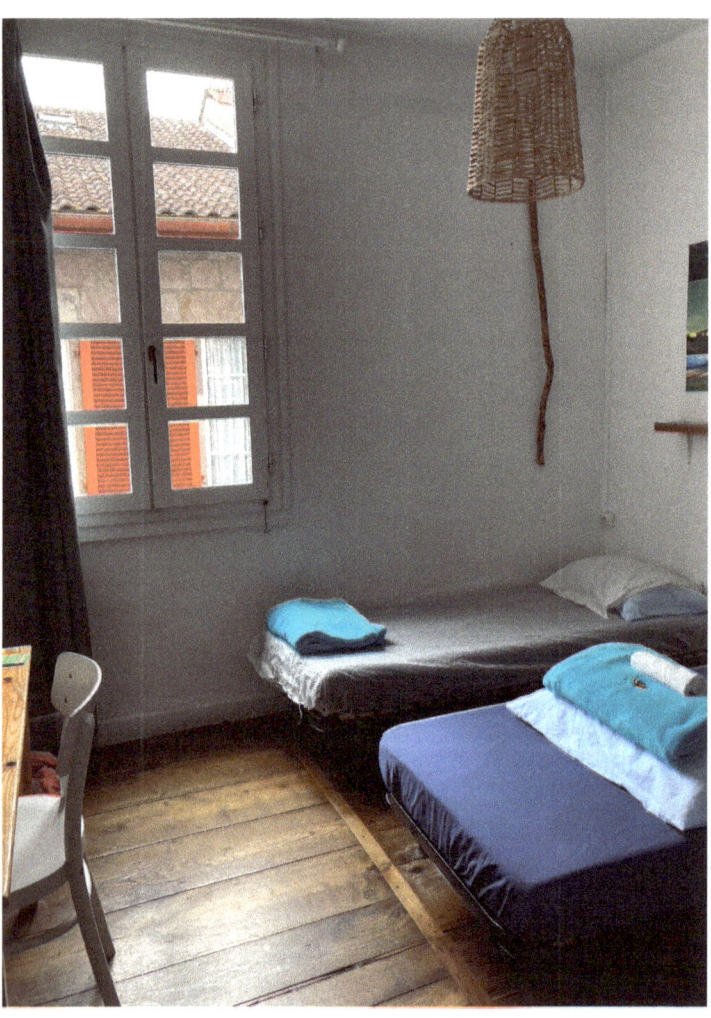

AVOIDING BEDBUGS

While not as disruptive as gastrointestinal distress, being attacked by bedbugs—not once but twice—was pretty darn awful. Yep, it's true. This happened to me. The bites are incredibly itchy and take many days to heal, and in the meantime are also terrible to look at. Yuck!

Of course, I had heard about bedbugs on the Camino, but just like I didn't think I'd have to take a bus and wouldn't get sick, I also didn't think bedbugs would apply to me!

Why? Because I believed I was taking the appropriate precautions. I was walking in a shoulder season, I had bought a silk sleeping sack, and I was using it in places I'd been told have the bugs—the dorms of the albergues. I would put my sleeping bag next to my skin and use the silk liner as a casing for me and the sleeping bag. I had no problem with bedbugs when I did this.

My mistake was not using the silk sack all the time. When I stayed in private rooms that had sheets, I mistakenly assumed these were "safe" and therefore abandoned the sleeping bag and silk sack. Wrong!

I also didn't know that you should always check any bed you are going to sleep in for signs of bedbugs. Look for small dark spots about the size of a bullet point symbol (this is their poop), pale yellow skins that are the shells the young ones shed, eggs that are yet to hatch, and of course live bedbugs. Do your research so you know what all of these look like!

And if you do end up with bedbug bites, it's a good idea to launder everything in your pack and dry it on a hot setting to make sure you're not carrying the little critters with you! For the bites themselves, try a cream that contains hydrocortisone or tea tree oil for the itching. And if you are prone to inflammation, consider taking an oral antihistamine to control any swelling of the bites.

EMBRACING PERSPECTIVE

I can't quite remember where I met Darya, in which town along the way. But I do know that it was in a church. And I know she was praying. I found out later, as we left the church together and struck up a conversation, that she was praying for peace and her whole country of Ukraine.

Listening to Darya talk about what life was like during a time of war and invasion was both eye-opening and devastating. It reminded me that you can never really know what someone else is living until you hear a personal account. Watching or hearing the news just doesn't cut it.

The Camino had dealt me a few blows, and I'd spent more than a minute feeling sorry for myself, but Darya's story quickly put everything in perspective. Our interaction shed light on the blessings of my life that I had been taking for granted. What a gift in that instant to have my own privilege and good fortune pointed out to me.

You are going to meet people from all over the world as you walk your path. This is simply a reminder to really listen to people's stories, put yourself in their shoes, and seize the chance to gain some perspective.

NEARING THE END

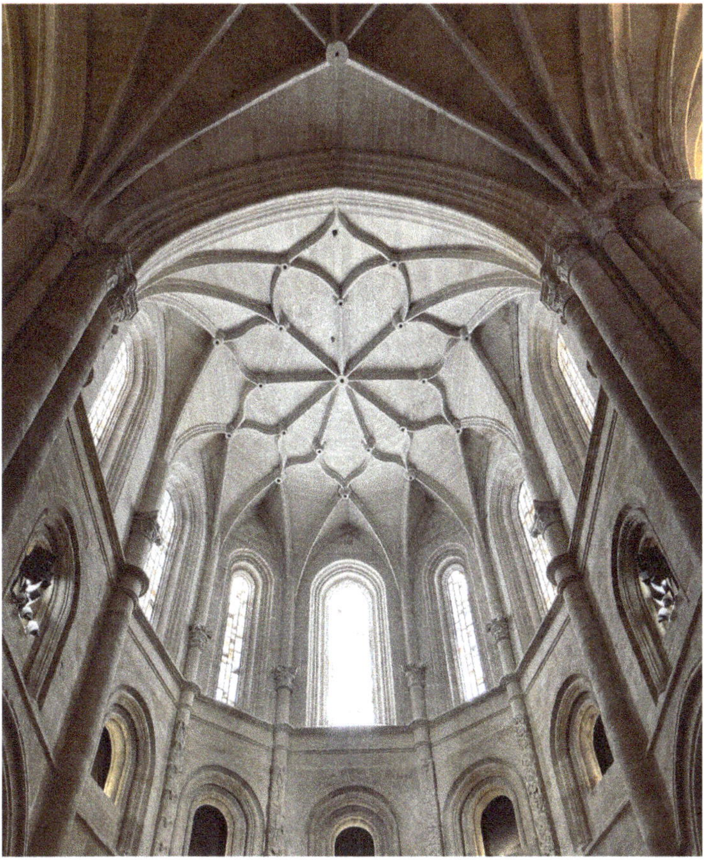

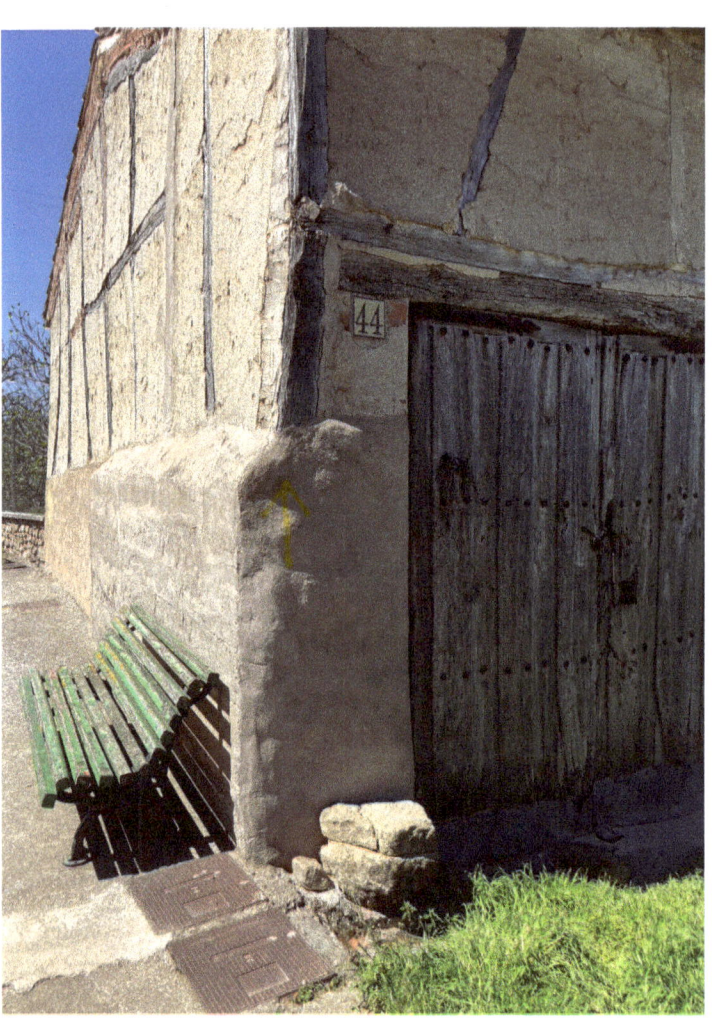

LETTING GO

I blame the haze of the heat and the haze of my illness for one of the decisions that I most regret on my Camino. Without anything but faulty intuition and my desire for a lighter pack to base my decision on, I decided to send home all the warm things I'd packed. Sadly, I didn't think to look ahead to the weather in the Galician region. Duh!

For an exorbitant amount of money, I sent home my winter hat, my long-sleeve shirt, my gloves, *and* my lightweight, puffy jacket. I almost mailed my rain jacket too, because I had the larger, newly purchased poncho for the rain but at the last minute decided to keep it. Thank God.

I didn't miss any of these items until the Meseta faded into the distance and I headed up into the mountains again. Right, the mountains! Higher altitude, colder temperatures. Damn. I heartily wished for every single item I had sent home. Why didn't I just trust my packing list and keep what I had decided on?

I'm not trying to dissuade you from sending things home that you might not need but rather to advise you that, like I've written before, you never really know what is going to happen and what you are going to need—in life or on the Camino!

While I wish I hadn't "let go" of all my warm clothes, letting go of emotional baggage is a different kettle of fish. We don't ever have to worry about sending that shit away and then missing it later!

As I mentioned in an earlier chapter, with the long stretches of road, plus the quiet and solitude that the Camino offers, you are going to have a lot of time to think. You may have helpful revelations about your life back home, but you may also have intrusive and painful thoughts or life regrets on rapid repeat.

The Camino Francés offers a place to release such emotional baggage. It's called Cruz de Ferro or the Iron Cross. It's a small hill, between the towns of Mandarin and Foncebadón, made up of stones, fluttering pieces paper and flags, with a huge cross on top. Many pilgrims carry a small stone with them to represent an emotional burden they would like to release. When they get to Cruz de Ferro, they leave the stone with the hope that they are also leaving the emotional baggage behind.

Give some thought to your own emotional burdens. Is there something you've been carrying with you—an old grudge or a hidden shame—that you'd like to leave behind on your Camino? Places like Cruz de Ferro are symbolic. Intellectually, we all know that we can leave any emotions, habits, or patterns of thought behind at any time. But there's something magical about a ritual we share as a community, one where we collectively choose to let something go that has been holding us back and walk into our future feeling lighter.

WALKING IN THE RAIN

As mentioned, I'd bought a special rain poncho in Saint Jean on the recommendation of a couple of people who'd walked the Camino before me. But after three plus weeks of no rain, I had been starting to think it was a waste of money. And then came Galicia. This lush, heavily forested region is roughly the last third of the Camino Francés, and it usually sees more rain than other parts of the path. Was I ever glad I had both the poncho *and* the raincoat!

You may have heard the adage: There is no such thing as bad weather, only bad gear. Well, I'm here to tell you it's true. Walking in the rain can be cozy and comfortable, and even beautiful, *if* you are dry.

Here are a few tips:

- Consider investing in a knee-length, waterproof poncho that is large enough to cover your backpack.

- I would suggest both a raincoat and a poncho! The raincoat is good for misty days and also acts as a shell for colder weather, while the poncho is excellent for the real downpours.

- To me, rain pants are an optional item, because if you wear a poncho, most of your body is going to be covered. I had a pair of lightweight hiking pants that I wore underneath the poncho, and they always dried quickly.

- I've seen debates about this on the Camino forums, but I was personally really glad that my footwear was waterproof. Many people choose to wear a sneaker or trail shoe because they are lightweight, but they definitely don't keep your feet dry and comfortable on massive rain days.

- As I mentioned, I sent my gloves home when I thought the heat was going to continue. But wow, were my hands cold on the rainy days! I would recommend a pair of lightweight, waterproof gloves.

- I didn't know such a thing existed, but in addition to waterproof boots or shoes, there are also waterproof socks! A friend I met on the Camino swore by them. Something to consider.

STAYING OPEN

As a person who is spiritual but not religious, I still enjoy exploring the deep quiet of Christian churches and feeling the energy of all the people who have knelt and prayed and sang there over time. It's a powerful and palpable feeling.

There is no shortage of churches along the Camino, some of which are grand and ornate, while others are simple, tiny stone structures. I poked my head into one of these on a rainy day, expecting the usual quiet, but was instead welcomed by both a priest and a nun seated at a table inside the door.

The nun led the conversation, and the priest translated. They asked where I was from and if I would like a pilgrim blessing (basically a prayer for a pilgrim's safe travel). I hadn't received one of these yet so gratefully accepted. Especially after being so sick, it felt like a no-brainer to receive a blessing for the remainder of the journey.

When I said yes, the tiny nun rose to her feet and came to stand in front of me. Holding a necklace with a pale blue string and a thin silver pendant, she stood on her toes to put it around my neck. Her worn hands were warm as she took mine, and then, looking directly into my eyes, she recited a prayer in Spanish. I had no idea what she was saying, but it didn't matter at all. A feeling of deep love washed over me and through me, causing tears to prick my eyes and warmth to flood my heart.

I met both Christians and non-Christians along the way, and one thing I noticed was that non-Christians weren't as keen to check out the churches. Like me, you might not be religious. And you might not be walking for any sort of religious or even spiritual reason. But the Camino *is* an ancient Christian pilgrimage route, and as such, there are a lot of churches, religious stories, and iconography.

Of course, you get to choose how much of that you would like to take in, but I think if we are open, we can receive the magic and miracles of any spiritual tradition, even if we don't belong to that tradition or claim it as our own.

Here's my perspective on what happened with the tiny nun in the quiet of that church. I think she sent me a shot of pure, undiluted love that my heart recognized and hungrily soaked up. While a Christian might call what I experienced "God's love," for me, it was just Love, with a capital *L*. And I don't think you have to be a Christian to feel its magical and palpable energy.

We humans have a tendency to shut the door on things that lie outside our comfort zones or stand in contrast to what we believe in. I want to encourage you to maintain an openness in your heart. You never know where and how love is going to show up as you walk your path.

SPEAKING YOUR TRUTH

As I've mentioned, you are going to meet some lovely people on your walk. People you really connect with and wish you could take home to be everyday friends. But the opposite is also true. Just like everywhere in life there are also boorish folks walking the Camino, the ones who can't read social cues and who stick to you even when you're trying to shake them off.

I was in the mountains again and really trying to soak it up after the monotony of the very flat Meseta, but the person who had somehow latched on to me was making that difficult. His voice was loud and grating, and he seemed perfectly content to monopolize the conversation. He hadn't asked me a single question! I felt invisible. Or more accurately, I felt I could be anyone. He wasn't engaging with me as another human being. He was just talking. Ad nauseam.

Having grown up in a culture where women are taught to be "nice girls" (polite even to assholes), I have always found it difficult to deal with situations like this. In not wanting to be rude, I have put up with other people's self-absorbed nonsense. In not wanting to hurt anyone else's feelings, I have stayed in situations that weren't serving me.

As my walking companion droned on, I reminded myself that this trip was my own and I didn't need to keep walking with someone I wasn't enjoying. So, on the outskirts of the next town where there were a series of benches, I screwed up my courage and decided to act. "I'm going to stop here and rest a minute. I'll see you down the road."

To my horror, he started to unbuckle his pack and moved to sit down, saying, "I'll wait for you." Foiled! It seemed I was being pushed to be even more clear and unequivocal.

I took a deep breath and rephrased: "Actually, I just really need some time alone." A look of confusion and then mild irritation crossed his face as I held firm.

"Fine. Whatever," he said and left, hurrying to catch up to another poor pilgrim who had just passed us. I patted myself on the back and felt a wave of relief wash through me. Not only did it feel good to be rid of Mr. Boorish, but I also felt proud that I'd listened and attended to what I needed.

I've talked to a lot of women about their impetus for walking the Camino, and many have said a version of this: "I've been taking care of others for a long time, and this is a trip that is just for me." Is that your story too?

If so, and if you are a caretaker and a people-pleaser by nature (as many of us are), you will need to stay connected to your own needs on this path and not get sidelined by other people's needs or desires.

I talked to one woman who had planned to do the walk on her own. She felt the solo journey was important to her, but within a few days had met someone who "stuck." They walked at a similar pace and had a lot in common. On one hand, it was wonderful to have a friend to walk with, and on the other hand, she wondered if she was missing out because her "alone time" was eclipsed.

There will likely be many days when—even if you are enjoying walking with someone else—one of you will end up needing or wanting something different: to walk a bit faster, to slow down, to stop for a break, or to have some alone time. Most people you'll meet are aware that this is the way of the Camino. Everyone is responsible for their own needs, and we all work at not being offended or hurt.

It's your trip, so you get to decide, but I recommend that you check in with yourself about what YOU really want on your journey. Your time on the Camino is precious, and it's also an excellent place to practise saying what you need.

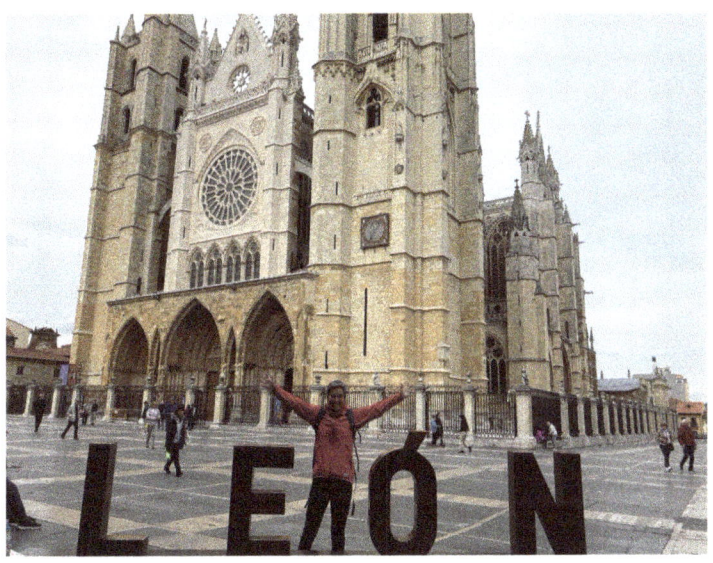

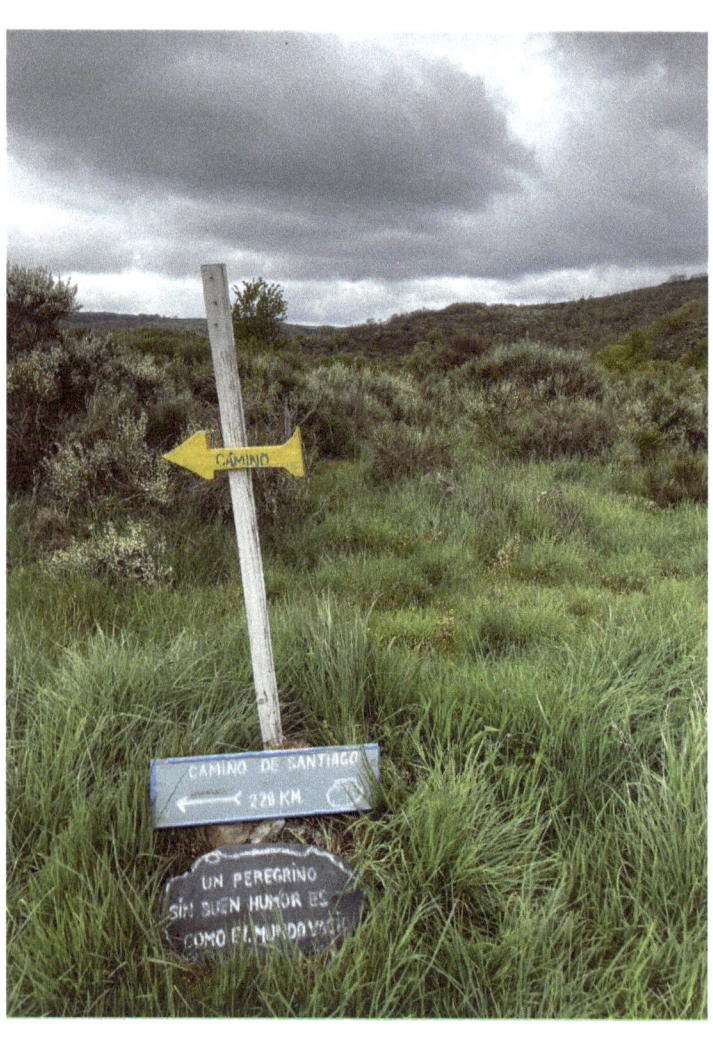

GOING WITH THE FLOW

Sometimes when something unexpected happens, or when things go off script, there is a beautiful result.

I was longing for some peace and quiet on the day I saw a small chalkboard sign outside a door: "Meditation at 6 p.m." On closer inspection, the building was a meditation studio, the first I had come across. I hustled off to the albergue where I was booked for the night, dropped my bag, and had a little rest.

A few hours later, I walked through the door of the studio, inhaled the scents of incense, fresh flowers, and herbal tea, and felt myself relax. The large room I had walked into was empty with no signs of a meditation happening. I spied a set of beautiful wide-plank wooden stairs leading to an upper floor and quietly walked up. There were three people: two folding up yoga mats, and one woman standing by the window and looking out.

"Is this where the meditation is?" I asked.

"Yes, usually," one of the two mat rollers said. "But I don't think there is one tonight."

I felt instantly disappointed and also confused. It wasn't clear if they worked there or were also there for the meditation, and I found out later that neither was true. They were pilgrims who had heard about the beautiful open space and used it to do some stretching and yoga. Good idea!

And then the woman at the window turned around and said: "I came for the meditation too." We struck up a conversation and ended up going back downstairs to discover a man filling tea carafes. He apologetically confirmed there was no meditation that evening. "But you're welcome to have a tea and enjoy the space."

My new friend, Jasmine, and I grabbed a tea and decided to take our conversation outside. We strolled down the streets of town before finding a bench with a lovely view.

It turned out to be one of those magical Camino conversations, with no small talk and where a connection is forged very quickly. In fact, Jasmine and I are still in touch and have a catchphrase for our friendship: "Best meditation we never went to!"

The lesson for me here was a simple one and one that I felt I learned repeatedly on the Camino. Don't be too attached to your idea of how things are going to go, or should go. Stay open to surprise. And delight.

DEALING WITH DISILLUSIONMENT

There may be days on the Camino—there certainly were for me—where the walk isn't measuring up to your expectations, or when you won't remember why you are doing it, or when you feel disillusioned with the Camino itself.

On the day I was nearing Sarria, only one hundred kilometres from the end of the path, I had a day like this. Ask any pilgrim and they'll tell you about the shift that happens around the Sarria mark. Suddenly there are way more people joining the path, and it starts to feel quite busy. Additionally, in this section of the Camino, I encountered some locals who seemed tired of dealing with pilgrims and where the Camino had the feeling of an industry rather than a spiritual pilgrimage.

So, I was feeling a bit jaded and deflated on the day I met Anat, a tour guide and ceramic artist from Israel. But after walking with her for only an hour, my whole outlook shifted. She was one of those people who paid attention, noticed the beauty around her, and remarked on it with awe.

Anat had just started walking a couple of days before and had an invigorating perspective on the beauty that was all around us, despite living in a home country that, at that time, was engaged in war. She was a breath of fresh air for me, and I inhaled deeply.

It's okay to become disillusioned. The Camino is many things—it IS an industry, it IS an economic driver, and it IS a way of life for some who live along the route, but it's also an ancient, sacred pilgrimage route where magic and epiphanies abound.

If you're having an off day, be kind to yourself. The best advice I can give you is to find a way to accept what is happening, rather than looking for what you wished for. And also remember to allow yourself the chance to be pulled away from the brink and back to the land of gratitude and wonder by the people you encounter.

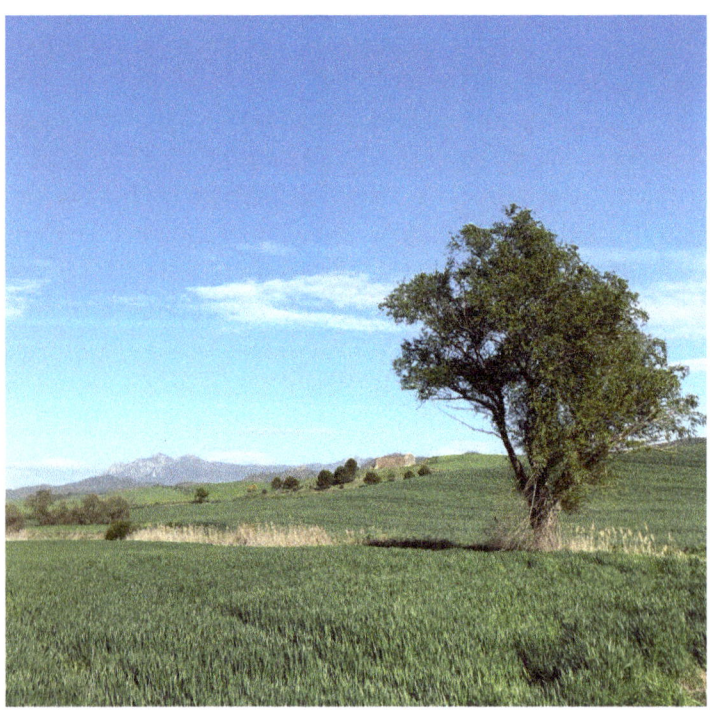

GIVING AND RECEIVING NEWS

The family and friends you leave behind are going to want to know how you are doing. They are going to want to see photos and hear stories. They might want to talk to you or see your face. And you might want this too! Give some thought to what kind of contact you feel would be best for you and the people you love while you are away on your big trip.

Before I left on my Camino, I had conversations with family about how we would keep in touch while I was away. My parents, my daughter, and my sister and I all got connected on WhatsApp to send photos and messages, and I was able to give them a phone number in Spain that came with the eSIM card I bought. We agreed that they would only call that phone number in an emergency and that we would use the free platforms of WhatsApp or FaceTime to connect otherwise.

My partner and I agreed to text at least twice a day—a good morning and a good night—and if I had time to send any messages during the day, great. We said we would also video call every once in a while, especially if one of us really needed support. What I didn't know was that she had also written out thirty postcards and put them in the post for me to receive at post offices all across Spain. I had my own unexpected cheering squad!

My biggest concern when I was away was my mother, who had been ill for a couple of months before I left. She was in recovery mode by the date of my departure, but with both of my parents in their eighties, I was a little worried about being so far away if I was needed. I definitely didn't want to receive that "bad news" call from home.

In the end, I did end up getting bad news from home, but it wasn't from my parents. It was an early morning call from my partner telling me that everyone was fine, humans and animals, but we had had a house fire. This news came three days from the end of my Camino, and I was faced with a tough decision: finish my walk or immediately return home.

I can only hope that you do not receive this kind of news, or any bad news, from home while you are walking your Camino. What I can tell you, having been through it, is that if you do receive bad news and have to make a difficult decision, there are people you'll meet on the Camino who will help and support you. I felt so lucky to have made such close friends prior to receiving news of the fire. All of these people, either through WhatsApp messages or in-person hugs, were there for me in the days after this devastating phone call from home.

ENCOUNTERING CAMINO ANGELS

In my Camino research over the years, I had heard the term "Camino Angel" over and over. Stories of someone appearing on the path when you most need help or a kindness. After walking the Camino now and encountering one myself, I can definitely say that they exist and their appearance does indeed seem magical.

Here's my story:

On the morning that I learned about our house fire and after anguished conversations with my partner, Malve, and my daughter, Sadie, I sat in the albergue, my head in my hands, not knowing what to do, even in the face of their unequivocal support.

"Mama, you've been wanting to do this for as long as I can remember," Sadie said. "You have to finish."

And from Malve: "There's nothing you can do, my love. I'll take care of things until you get home. It's only a few days. Please finish your walk. I know how much it means to you."

But with such a massive event that would cause so much disruption, it seemed wrong, and somehow selfish, to not immediately return home. As I got dressed, I resolved to use the day ahead of me to decide whether to end my trip and return home early.

As I left the albergue and walked out of town, I whispered a prayer for guidance. "Please put someone on my path today who will help me get through the day and make this tough decision."

Within minutes (I'm not kidding), I met Mary and learned she was from Halifax, my home city. If this had been the only sign that Mary was a Camino Angel it would have been enough. It felt like a miracle to meet someone from home, and it immediately caused me to burst into tears and tell her about the fire. She hugged me close and cried with me. Another miracle.

And then, as if the universe needed to make sure I got the message that Mary had been divinely placed on my path, she pulled something from her waist bag. In order to understand the significance of what I am about to tell you, here is a little backstory.

Every morning from the time Sadie was quite small, we had a morning ritual over breakfast. We pulled an "angel card" to start our day. These are small cards that I'd bought and placed in a pottery bowl, each with its own word: Tenderness. Grace. Love. Spontaneity. Joy.

Sadie had creased the ones she loved the most so that when she closed her eyes and felt around in the bowl, she would know which ones to pick. So much for allowing the divine to provide a daily message! In the time since Sadie grew up and moved out, Malve and I have continued the morning ritual, choosing an angel card to set the tone for the day.

Yep, you guessed it. Mary had angel cards in her belt bag! That morning, she offered me a card and then walked with me for the next four hours, matching the lethargy of my shocked and reeling pace, listening closely, and gently offering words of empathy and wisdom.

By the end of our time together, I knew I would finish what I had started. I would complete my long walk and then return home where a whole new journey would unfold.

The angel card I chose? Resilience.

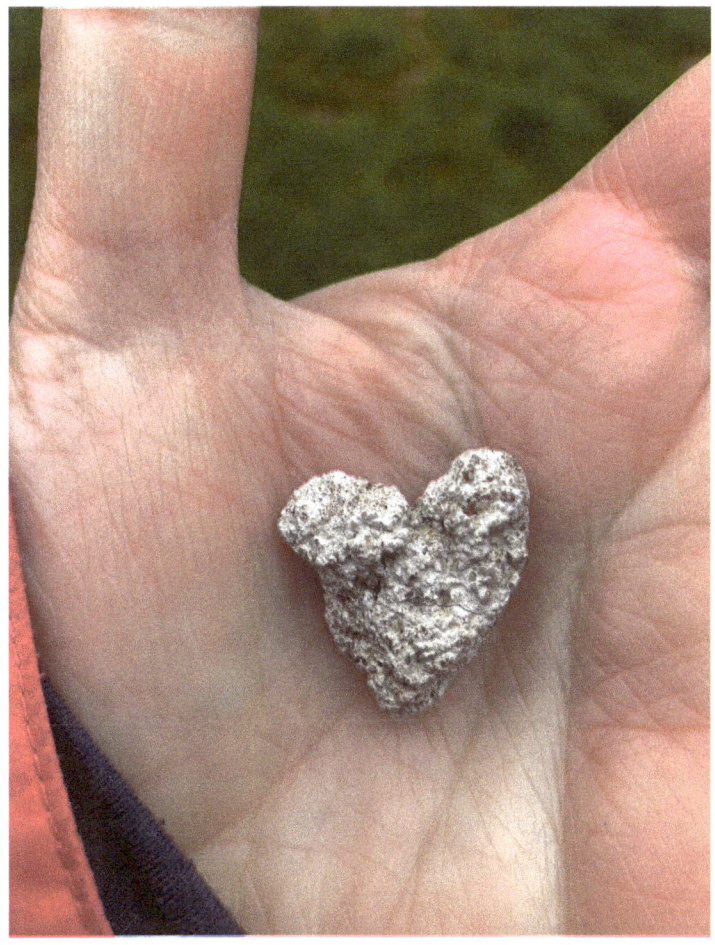

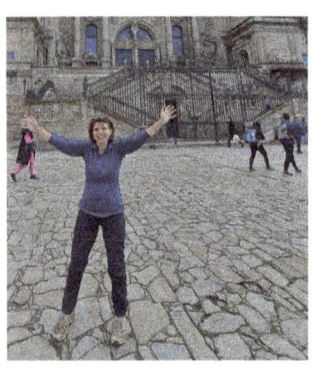
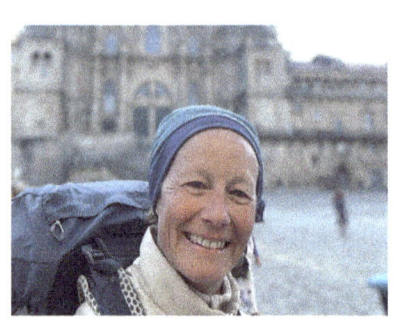
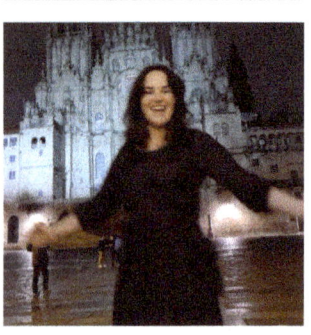
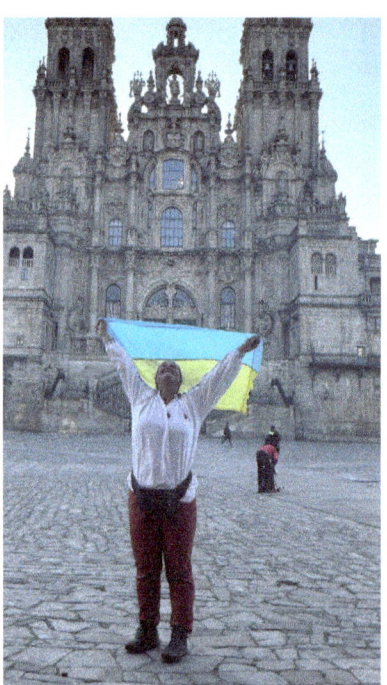
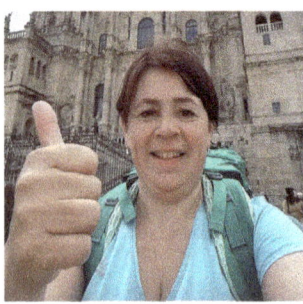

FINISHING YOUR SOLO CAMINO

Most of the Camino routes through Europe end in the same place—at the historic cathedral in Santiago de Compostela, in a large public square called the Plaza de Obradoiro.

Walking into the square, knowing you are taking the last steps of your Camino, is powerful stuff. It's also a little surreal. The trip you may have been planning for years is officially over, and you will likely be filled with different emotions.

I had literally spent years imagining a "hallelujah" moment as I walked through Santiago at the end of my long journey and the cathedral came into sight. I fantasized about the feelings that would fill me, that thrilling sense of pride and accomplishment, and the tears that would flow because I had done it. And I had done it on my own.

But just like in life, things don't always turn out the way you planned. After the news of our house fire and the appearance of my Camino Angel, I continued on. However, when I look back on it now, those last few days are a bit of a blur. I did have the moment of entering Santiago, dropping my bag in the cathedral square, and bursting into tears, but it felt much different than I had imagined.

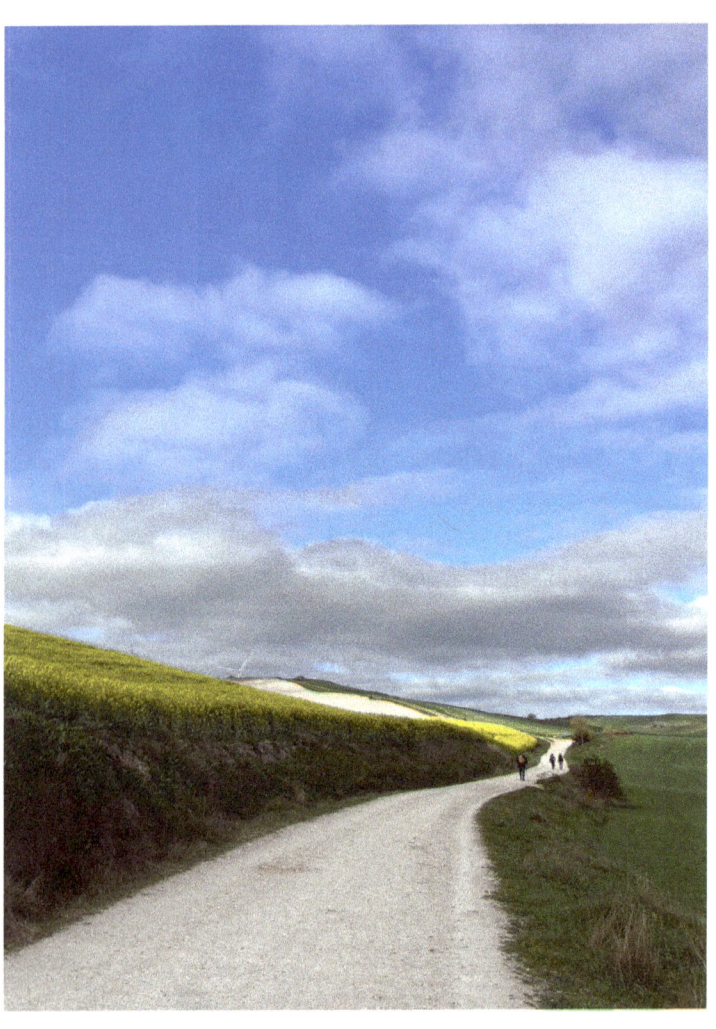

FINISHING YOUR SOLO CAMINO

Just like your whole Camino experience, the culmination of your journey will be uniquely your own. You may raise your hands in the air and have someone snap a photo of you in the ultimate victory pose. Or you may drop to the ground in exhaustion.

Wherever, and whenever, your trip ends, be kind to yourself. Endings are often hard, so take good care of yourself and respect what you need. If it's possible, give yourself some time to both rest and decompress after you finish walking. What you will have accomplished is no small feat, either physically or emotionally, and you may need some time and space to process and integrate your experiences.

That's what we'll cover in the next section!

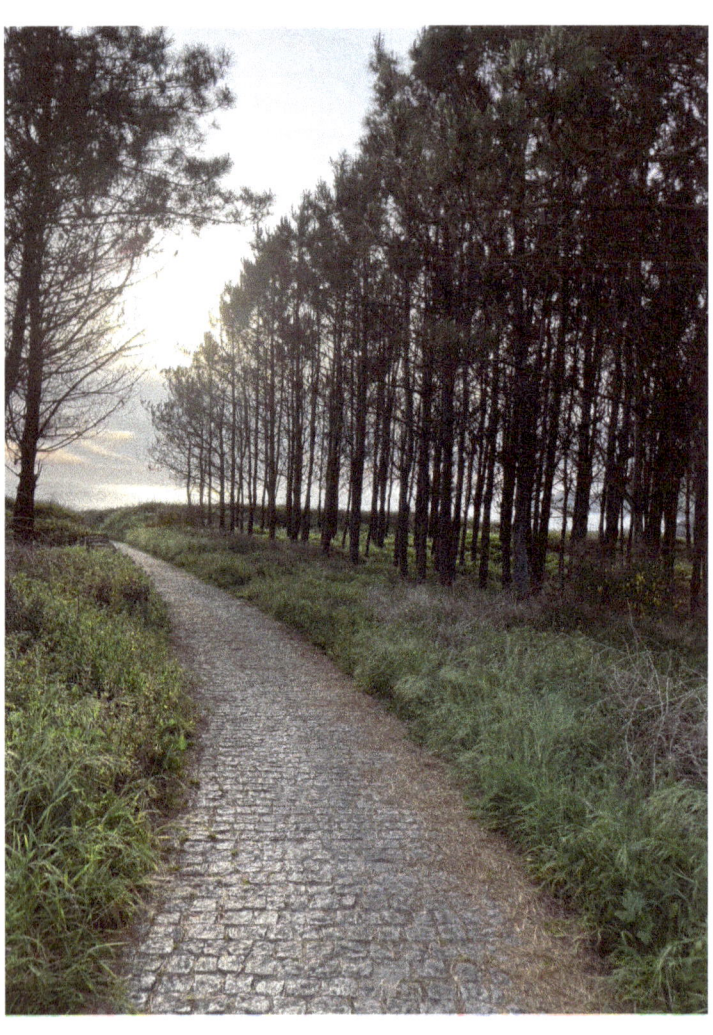

PART FOUR

THE PATH CONTINUES: AFTER YOUR CAMINO

Some people say their lives changed after walking the Camino. Other people say it was a fun and interesting way to spend a month or six weeks. Still others say the whole thing didn't live up to the hype.

Every single one of us who chooses to walk the Camino has both a different reason for wanting to do it and also a unique experience of walking it. No two are ever the same. The way we end up framing or summarizing the whole trip is also hugely individual. You get to decide the stories you tell about it—to yourself and to others.

The truth is that life goes on after the Camino. But before the tide of your return sweeps you away, I'd like to encourage you to be as intentional, mindful, and kind to yourself as possible. That's what this section is about.

There are also lots of prompts for reflection and writing in this section that I encourage you to return to after your walk!

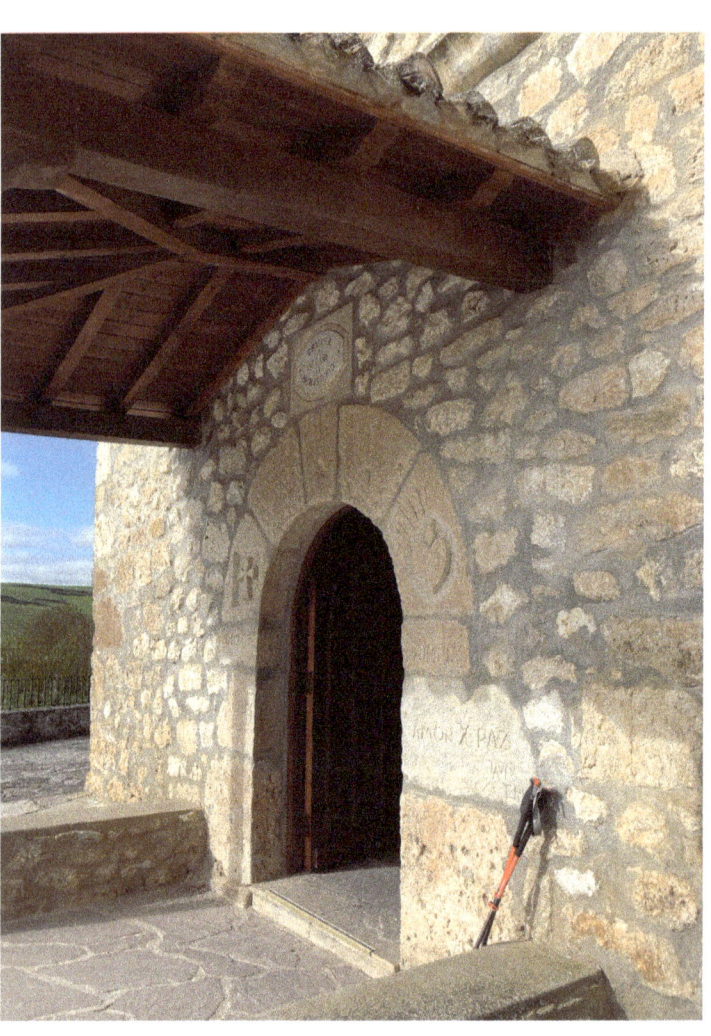

INCLUDING BUFFER TIME

Returning home can be rough after any kind of trip; sometimes there is a "deflation" period where you may struggle with low spirits or motivation. This might sound familiar if you've ever returned from a tropical vacation to a cold, grey winter! But after a long, involved, and intense adventure like the Camino, there is an even greater likelihood of re-entry bumps.

For one thing, you'll have just spent a month or more mostly outside. This daily experience is in great contrast to the lives most of us live: inside for work and home, with maybe an hour or a two a day getting exercise or moving from point A to B.

There is also the fact that on the Camino, no two days are ever the same! Every day a new place, every minute a fresh step. That's a lot of stimulation and variety, and with no set routine like most of us have at home. This "on the move" lifestyle can become addictive, and you might miss it once you return to the place where you live. On the other hand, you might be more than happy to come home to some predictable and ordinary patterns!

When you're planning your return home, do yourself a favour and block off a few days. I know this won't be possible for everyone, but if you can make it work (perhaps by arranging to arrive back home on a Thursday or Friday but not go back to regular routines until Monday), you will definitely benefit.

Here's why I am recommending a slow re-entry once you return home:

- If you have gotten used to being on your own and are now returning to the demands of family, it may be a shock to your system. A few extra days gives your body time to rest and your spirit space to adjust to being responsible for other people and their needs again. Especially if you are going back to a busy job or a caretaking role with children, aging parents, etc.

- This kind of "in-between" space, where your Camino is over but you're not quite back to the daily grind, is a way to honour your trip and to attend to anything that might need to be mulled over or savoured. The integration of all you may have learned or discovered on your trip won't happen overnight, but granting yourself a few days will help in the long run!

- If you live with other people, this buffer time will also help them. It's a way of "landing" and slowly reintegrating into home life and routines. This will ensure there isn't still a part of you that has remained in the country you walked through! Giving yourself the space to return from such a huge trip, in body and in spirit, is actually a gift to the people around you—your partners, children, friends, or workmates—all of whom will want to hear your stories and also share their stories with you!

SEEKING MEANING

When you're walking, you're often thinking about your sore feet or where you should stop for lunch or how many more kilometres there are to go. There isn't always the spaciousness to be able to feel an overall sense of significance or meaning.

But this kind of a long walk, especially when you do it alone, does have the potential to change you. It may reorder your priorities, it may refocus you on what's important, it may even change your idea of how you want to live.

That's why when you return, before the tide of your "now" life has a chance to carry you away, it's important to do some of your own meaning-making.

Consider building some time for reflection into your back-at-home schedule. This could be a few scheduled sessions where you look at your photos, relive your Camino, and perhaps put pen to paper to explore your experience.

I would recommend a daily practice, right after you return, where you sit down for twenty or thirty minutes before the day begins—perhaps with a morning cup of tea or coffee—and really immerse yourself in your Camino. I would do this for as long as it feels right to do so. You might never stop!

REFLECTION / WRITING PROMPTS:

What did your Camino mean to you?

What do you feel you gained? What are you grateful for?

How are you different from before you started walking?

What new things did you learn about yourself? What epiphanies or realizations did you have?

Are there things in your life you decided you wanted to change as you were walking? If so, what are they?

Are there any promises or commitments you want to make to yourself for your re-entry into life at home?

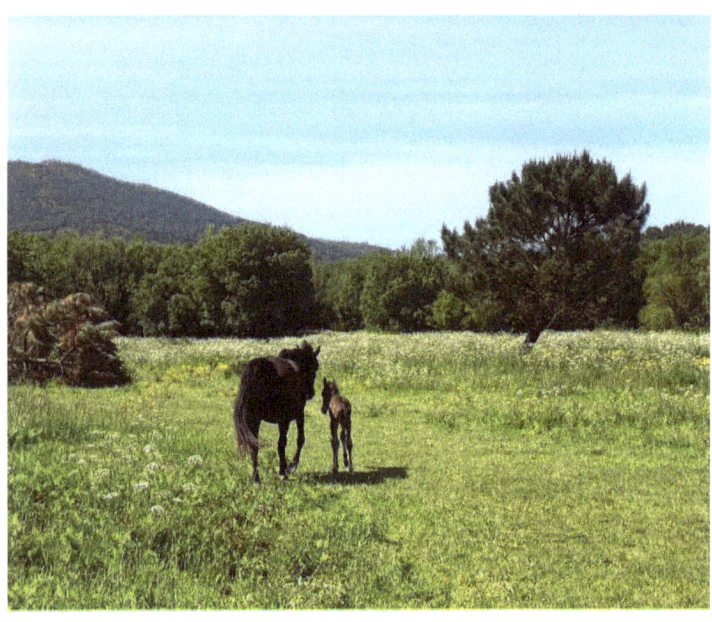

DEALING WITH CONTRADICTORY EMOTIONS

Just as everyone's actual Camino is different, so too are everyone's feelings about their Camino. Your emotions might feel complex and even contradictory during the first few days or weeks after returning. You may be excited to return home but miss the pace of life on the Camino and the new friends you made. You might be relieved to have completed the arduous walking part of the journey but don't necessarily want to go back to "real life."

In addition, your Camino might not have lived up to your expectations or hopes and you may be dealing with disappointment or regret. On the other hand, you might be super excited and want to hop back on a plane and do it all again.

You may have come to some new realizations but are unsure how you will incorporate what you have learned now that you're back. And if you did the Camino alone, you might really be missing your space and independence even though you're excited to be back home.

These big feelings or your conflicting emotions are all normal! Allow for all your feelings, and give yourself space for your realizations, your unanswered questions, your confusion, and all of your wonderings.

REFLECTION / WRITING PROMPTS:

What are your primary, or obvious, emotions? Are there others under the surface? Describe them.

Are you judging any of your feelings?

Is there a way you can be kind to yourself and allow for all the emotions that are present?

ACCEPTING YOUR UNIQUE CAMINO

No matter how much you read about or researched the Camino, it's impossible to know how your trip will unfold. Until it does.

During the last week of my trip, I reconnected with some of the people who were at that first pilgrim supper in Saint-Jean-Pied-de-Port. As we walked and talked, we marvelled at our naivety as we began the walk and struggled with the notion that our expectations hadn't quite matched up to our experience. One of my friends said something like, "If any of us write a book, we should call it 'Shattered Expectations'!"

It's a funny title (or at least we thought so!), but what *does* happen when the end result is something radically different than what you envisioned?

As I mentioned in Part Two, the WHY of my trip was to learn to trust myself more deeply and to provide for my own sense of safety while walking. That was why it was important to do the Camino on my own.

But what I didn't realize was that there was another expectation that was running parallel to this one and that went unexamined in the lead-up to my walk. I blame the movie *The Way*. And also all the books and online resources and podcasts where the idea of a "Camino family" is presented as an inevitable occurrence.

This deep-rooted expectation was that I would meet like-minded people and we would form a "Camino family," walking together every day and staying in the same places.

Now that I've walked the Camino, I know that in order for this to happen, the stars must align perfectly. You need to meet people who walk the same pace as you, want to walk the same distance as you, and want to stay in the same places as you. Every day for over a month!

The reality for me was that I met amazing people, but we didn't walk together for more than a few hours. For the first few weeks, I found this quite disappointing, and my inner critic was quick to point out that I must be doing something wrong.

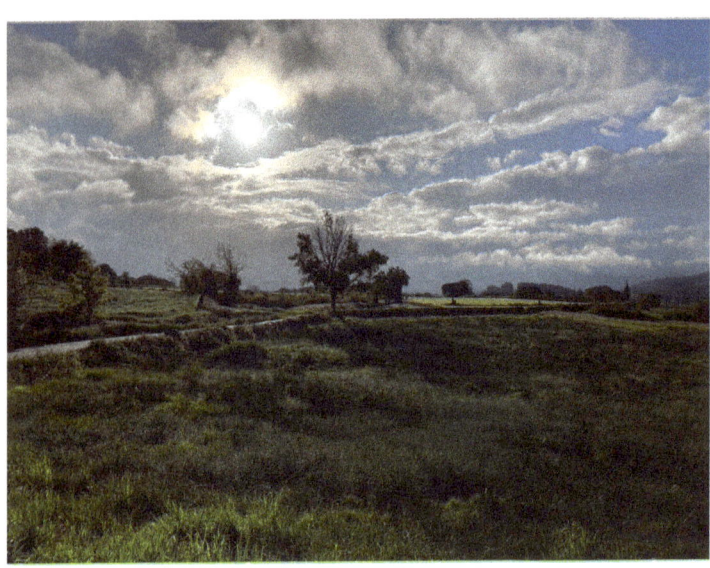

ACCEPTING YOUR UNIQUE CAMINO

But what I can clearly see now is that the only way I could learn to trust myself was to travel alone. I needed to make decisions by myself and for myself. I needed to provide my own sense of safety. Therefore, a Camino family was out of the question.

If you are grappling with your own "shattered expectations," know that you're not alone. And I hope you won't be too hard on yourself if you end up having a very different Camino than the one you thought you would!

REFLECTION / WRITING PROMPTS:

Did your Camino measure up to, exceed, or fall short of the expectations you had going into it? Give lots of details.

Are you feeling sad about any aspects of your trip? If so, is there anything you can offer yourself that will help you come to terms with any residual disappointment?

Even if your trip wasn't exactly as you envisioned, can you see now, with the benefit of hindsight, the ways you might have grown?

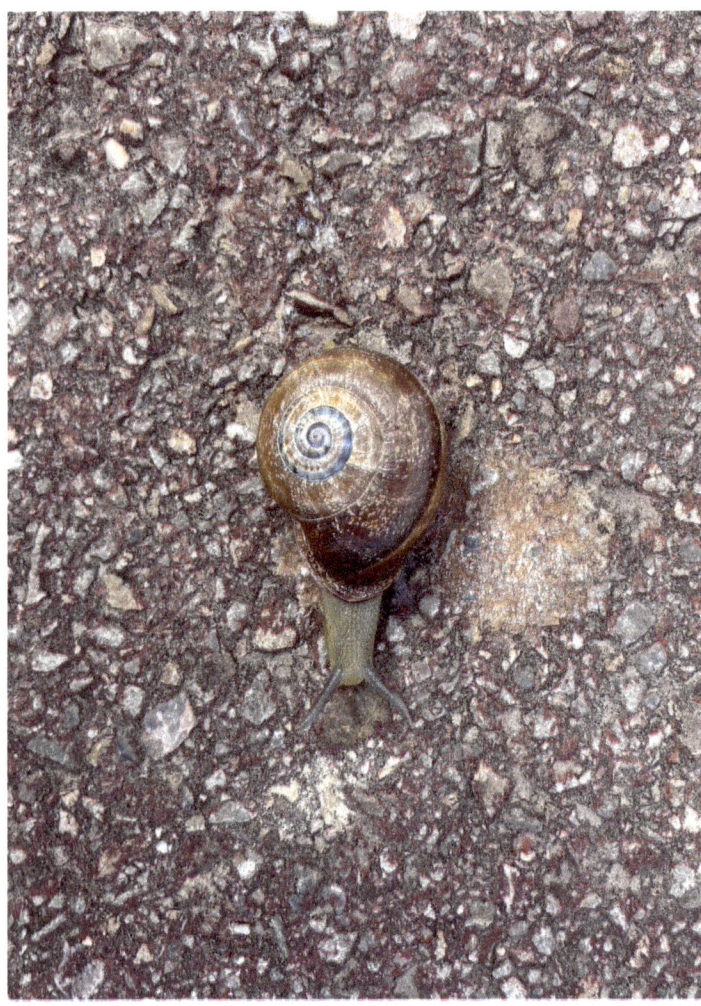

PRACTISING PATIENCE

Some pilgrims arrive home thinking nothing much happened for them. While this is possible, there is also a chance that what you gained from the trip may be parcelled out slowly upon your return.

Be patient with this. Sometimes the benefits or the learning of a trip like the Camino unfold gradually over time as we begin returning to normalcy and routines. Remember, you've been living in a very unusual state for the time you've been away—on the move constantly, with new people, experiences, sights, and sounds every day.

When you return home, and things calm down, you may notice that there have been changes inside you that you hadn't noticed while you were walking. You might feel calmer or stronger or more grounded in situations that used to make you feel undone. You may feel differently about a person or a job or a hobby or a pastime. You might have new ideas or dreams, or you may suddenly desire a change you didn't see coming.

While these realizations may not have risen to the surface on the Camino, that doesn't lessen their importance.

Wait for it! You might be in for a slow reveal.

REFLECTION / WRITING PROMPTS:

Are there any subtle changes you are beginning to notice in yourself?

Are your memories or ideas about the Camino, or things you thought you learned while walking, changing the longer you are home?

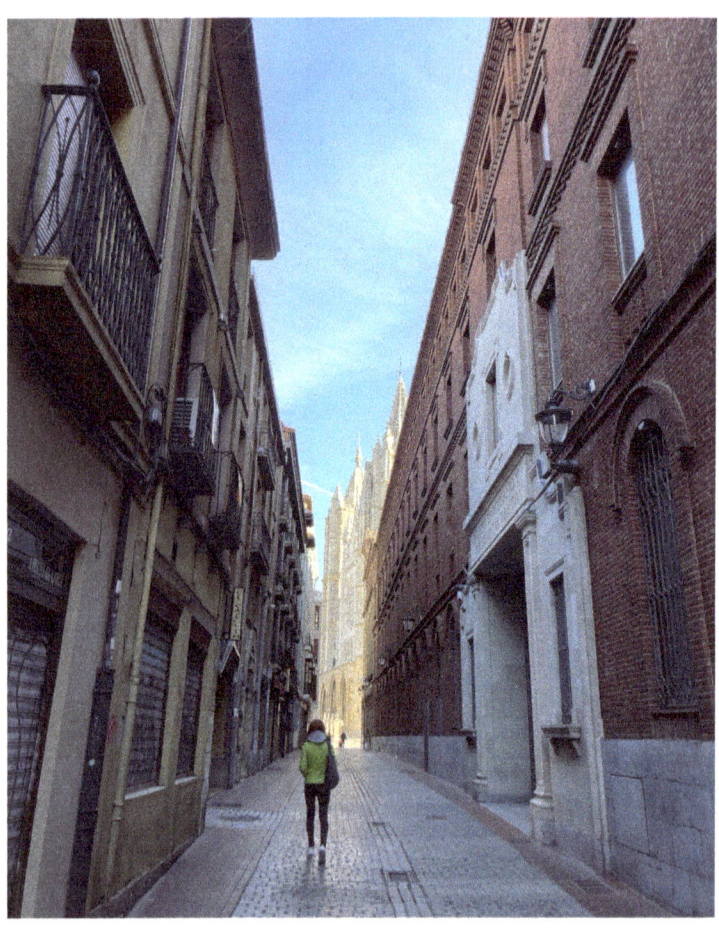

SHARING YOUR CAMINO

When we choose to walk the Camino, it can be a real community experience. Over the course of our preparation and training, we usually end up telling a lot of people—family and friends, of course, but also neighbours, gym buddies, workmates, and even the mail carrier—about our upcoming adventure.

Therefore, when you return, anyone who knew you were going to walk the Camino is going to want to know how it went. Be prepared!

The stories you tell about your Camino are very personal. There will be the story you tell in your own heart to yourself; the story you tell one or two of your closest family or friends; and the story you tell everyone else.

All of these stories require crafting, which also requires time. This might sound strange—I have to figure out what I am going to say to everyone?—but here's why.

It's a big trip in more ways than one. It's not only long, but it's intense, both physically and emotionally, and maybe spiritually. Coming up with a summary, especially for someone who has not had a Camino experience themselves, is very tricky indeed.

When I returned from mine, most people didn't ask me about it because our house fire was first and foremost on everyone's mind. And I have to say that I was a little bit relieved. I was already sensing that it would be impossible to fit the whole trip, with all of its complexities and contradictions, into an easily digestible sound bite.

I didn't want to cheapen my Camino by creating a summary version, and I was worried that I couldn't possibly do the whole trip justice. I was certain that, in trying to find all the right words, I would fail, and it would somehow diminish my experience.

Here are some ideas and options for you to consider when you return home and are grappling with how to talk about your Camino and what kind of story to tell:

- Go with the path of least resistance and give a one-word answer—"great" or "challenging" or "inspiring" or "epic"—and then leave it to the other person to ask specific questions that might be a little easier to field.

- Tell them you are still processing the trip and aren't ready to talk about the details quite yet. Bookmark the conversation until another time. If they ask again, you'll be more prepared.

- Consider an "elevator speech" of sorts. I came up with a short description of my journey that didn't full encapsulate everything but was also truthful and didn't diminish my experience. "It was ALL the things you can think of—hard, amazing, beautiful, painful, fascinating. And I met some absolutely incredible people."

- Use the photos you took, in lieu of words or in addition to words. Go through photos in the early days of your return home and choose a handful that really represent the feeling of the trip for you. A special sunrise? A communal dinner? You on top of a mountain? You with a friend? The pic of you in the cathedral square, arms raised in victory? Have them in a special photo folder on your phone; then when someone asks how your trip was, you can quickly show them.

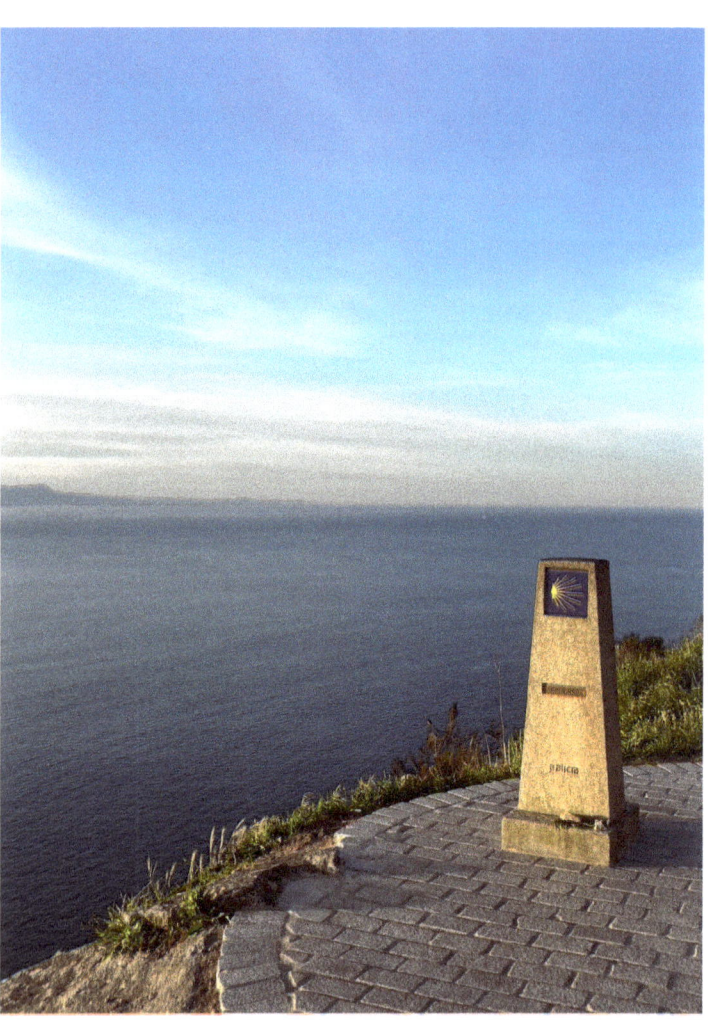

CELEBRATING YOURSELF

In Santiago, I took my last steps of the Camino. I hugged a few friends, I took some photos, I stood in line for my Compostela, and then I sat down and cried. My walk was over and almost immediately my mind turned to all that lay ahead: getting to the airport in Portugal, flying home to Malve's arms, and the enormity of our reality, post-fire.

But I had one last task. Finding the post office to retrieve the final postcard from Malve. I walked to the *Correos* office, said my line in Spanish—*Tienes correo para mi?*—and watched the employee disappear into the back. When she returned, she had not one postcard, but a whole stack of mail. I thought she'd gotten my name wrong, but as she passed me the pile and I started to go through it, every envelope was addressed to me! She grinned and gave me a thumbs-up as she watched my smile grow and grow.

Little did I know, Malve had asked my family and friends to send a card or letter of congratulations to Santiago so that I would feel well and truly celebrated when I finished my long walk. (I know, she is amazing!) She had planned this weeks before so all of the messages were written before the fire. This ended up being a real godsend, because the words I read that day—which made me feel so special and so seen—were purely about my Camino and not eclipsed in any way by the other major event.

Those notes did something for me that I wasn't able to do for myself at that time. They returned me to the present. For a few minutes that day, as I read and cried over those beautiful cards and letters, I was able to really feel the magnitude of what I had done. My friends and family saw my walk as an accomplishment, and as they celebrated it, so did I.

This is what I want you to do too. I want you to celebrate yourself and your Camino. No matter what happened along the way, no matter what news you received from home, no matter if it unfolded as you intended or went completely sideways.

Celebrate in whatever way feels right to YOU. By yourself. With others. Quietly. Loudly. With a party. Using a slideshow. Be intentional about it and find a way, or ways, to honour the enormity of what you have done.

This trip that you initiated, planned, prepared, and completed. This trip that was just for you. That you did all on your own. By yourself—for you, by you.

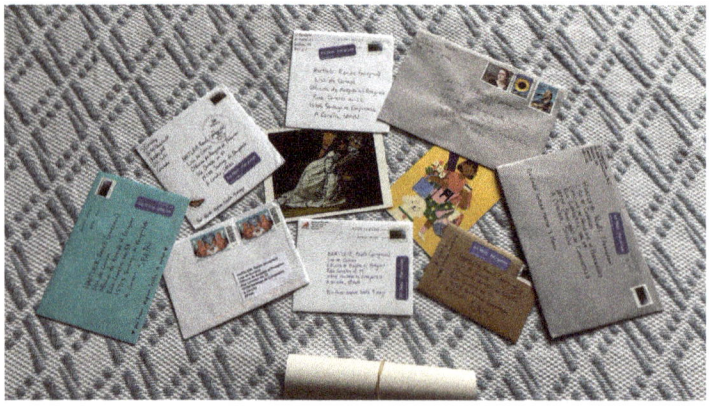

PLANNING THE NEXT ONE!

If this was your first solo trip, don't stop here!

Run with the momentum and begin planning your next adventure. Where does the thread want to lead you? Perhaps it's another pilgrimage. Or maybe a retreat. Or has a friend you made on the Camino asked you to visit them? Even if it's not a travel adventure, stay open to what else your heart is calling for.

REFLECTION / WRITING PROMPTS:

What did the Camino open up for you?

What are your thoughts about next steps?

What else is calling to you now?

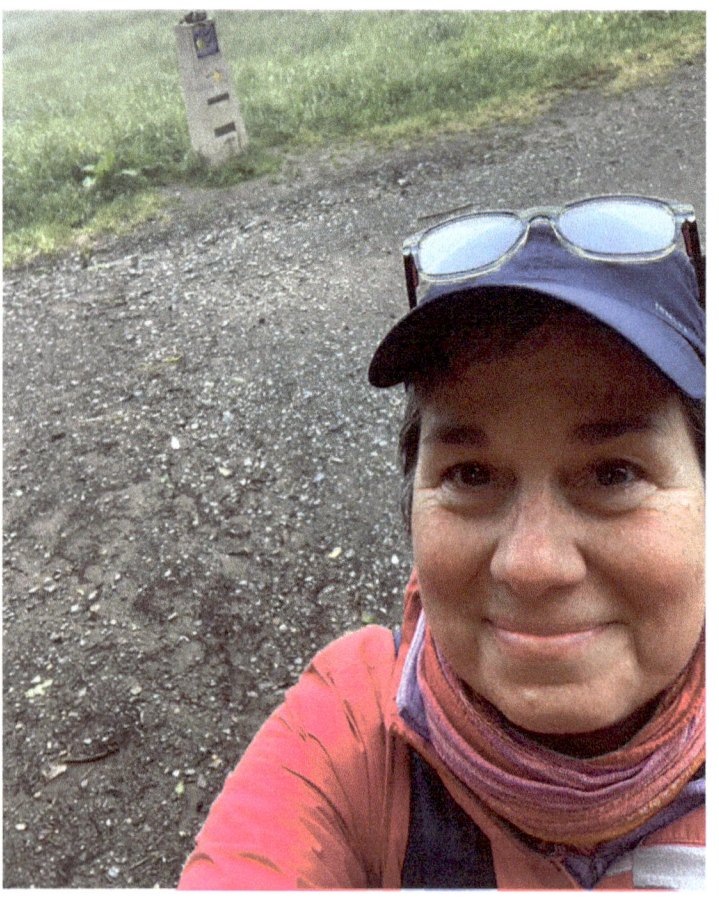

IN CLOSING

I truly hope that the words and stories I've shared in this book help you to believe in yourself and your abilities. And that they assist you in feeling prepared—mentally, physically, and emotionally—for the journey that lies ahead.

If you truly desire a solo trip, you can absolutely make it happen. Having done it myself, I can guarantee that you are stronger and more capable than you think. And you *deserve* to fulfill this dream.

As you close the pages of this book, I hope you experienced some "aha!" moments, chuckled at some of my missteps, and are moving into your upcoming adventure feeling inspired and enthused.

I urge you to remember that there is no one *right* way to do the Camino, that your best laid plans may just go off the rails, and that disappointment is normal. Please be kind to yourself in every and all situations. Your Camino will be unique and individual—yours and yours alone.

On a personal note, writing this book has been my way of dealing with the deep grief of losing our home. Every day during the demolition and rebuilding process, I've written and rewritten and edited the words you've been reading, and this has been my way of celebrating and reliving my Camino. The belief that my book would end up in the hands of the women who need it has been my beacon of light through a dark time.

Thank you for letting me accompany you. If you feel so inclined, I would love to hear how your Camino went and if my book helped you. Specifics and stories are very welcome!

renee@reneehartleib.com

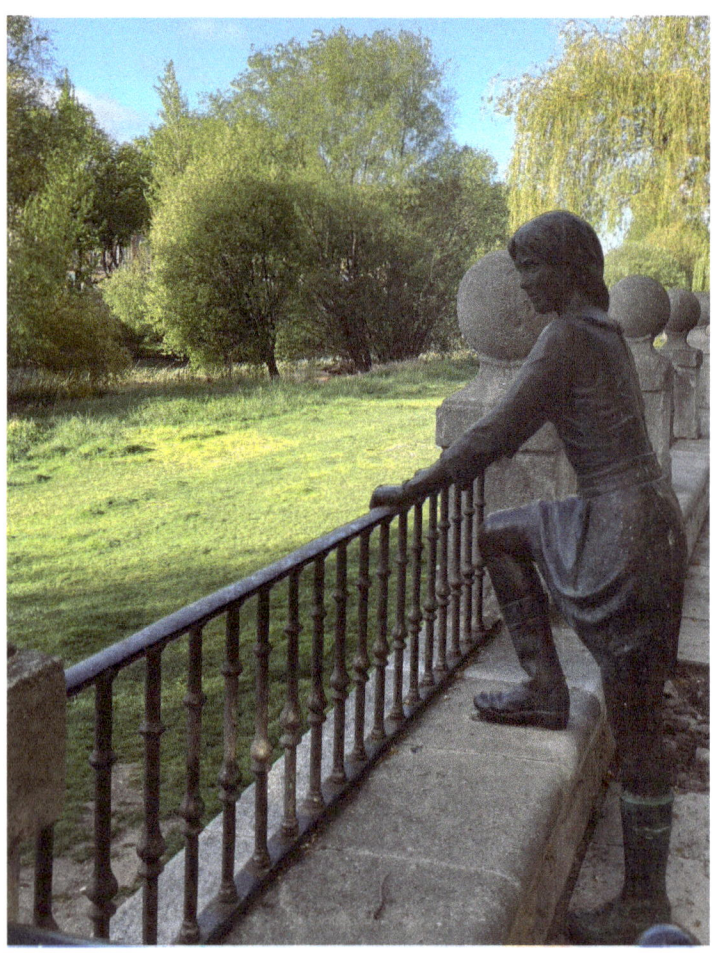

SPREAD THE WORD

Word of mouth is how news travels on the Camino. It's also the best way to spread the joy of a good Camino book. If you enjoyed my book and found it helpful, please tell your friends, family, neighbours, and walking clubs!

If you purchased my book off of Amazon, leave stars, or better yet, a short review. Glowing reviews and five-star ratings will help other women who want to do solo walks find my book!

Lastly, if you are interested in learning more about self-discovery and inner journeys, check out my first book, *Writing Your Way: A 40-Day Path of Self-Discovery.* And if you'd like to read more of my writing, go to my website: reneehartleib.com.

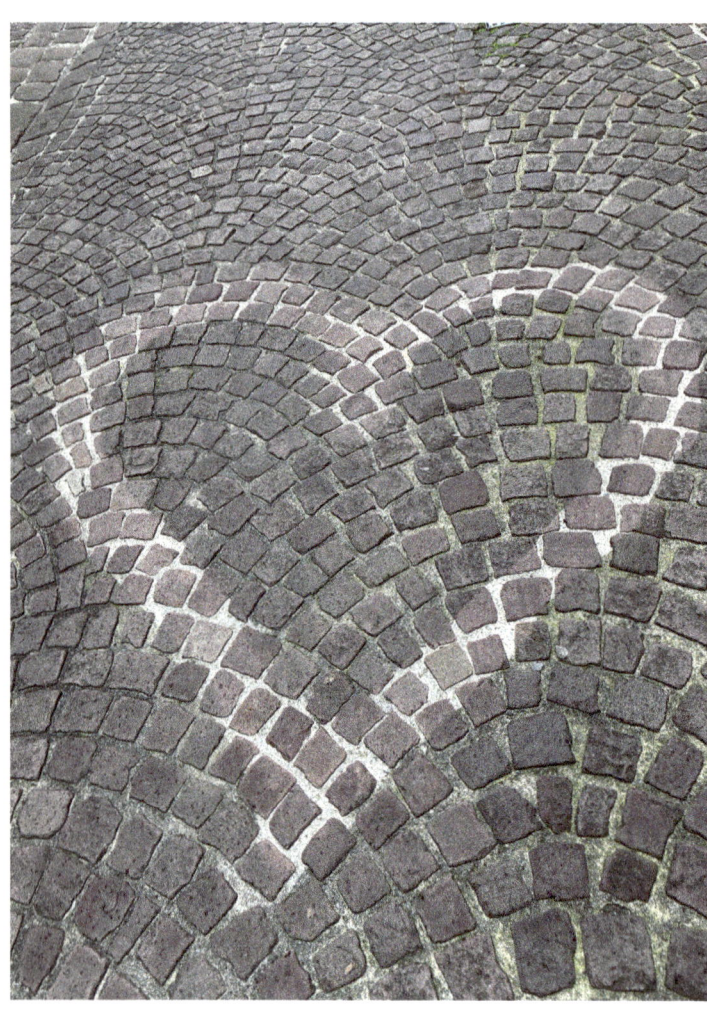

GRATITUDE

To my partner, Malve, always my first reader, for your belief in me and my book ideas and also for your love and support as I write them. And for your encouragement to go on my big Camino adventure—you were with me every step of my way.

To my other invaluable readers and friends, Maggie, Elisa, and Jasmine, for the enormous gift of your time and efforts, for your great ideas, for helping improve my sentences, and for your kindness and enthusiasm about my book!

To my parents and my sister for believing in me as a writer from way back when, for always asking how the book is coming along, and for celebrating with me now that it's out there!

To my daughter, Sadie, for inspiring me with your seeking and your travels and your independence, and for your love.

To Emmet and Esja, for your humour and kindness and for lightening these last many months in our home away from home.

To my wonderful writing group, Maggie, Jessie, and Elizabeth. Our evenings of food, laughter, and sometimes tears are a true balm.

To Janice and Claudette for sharing your home with me when I became office-less due to the fire and needed space to write this book. Your generosity knows no bounds, and I'm so humbled to benefit from the motto you truly live by: *Mi casa es su casa*.

To our Helping Hands Community of Halifax/Dartmouth who supplied meals, put IKEA furniture together, and supported our family after the fire, freeing up space for me to write this book.

To Marianne for your editing expertise and your friendship, to Megan for your kindness, patience and design talent, and to Sarah E. for our conversations about writing and your unflagging support.

To the owners, organizers, and women writers of Birchdale for your support and company as I finished a first draft of this book.

And in addition to Elisa and Jasmine (my Camino friends mentioned above), I am sending love and hugs to these wonderful souls I met on my Camino. Once strangers, now friends: Kellie, Peter, Priscila, Marcela, Petra, Darya, Eleanor, Laura C., Laura K., Nicole, Mark, Sofie, Anne, Colette, Amy, Mary, Darnell, Maxime, Jackie, Christine, Walli, Enrica, Luca, Jimmy, Beate, Kay, and Anat.

All photos have been taken by the author who holds the copyright, except for photos on page 96 supplied by Hyungjin Choi (top left), Marcela Aguilera (top middle), Peter Fredsholm (middle right), and Elisa Troyer (bottom right), plus photos on page 166 supplied by Petra Timmers (top left), Sofie De Mey (top right), Amy Twigg-Edwards (middle left), Enrica Colombi (bottom left), and Darya Dmytruk (middle right).

RESOURCES

Please check out the "Camino" section of my website for information, resources, and photos.

https://reneehartleib.com/camino

www.ingramcontent.com/pod-product-compliance
Lightning Source LLC
Chambersburg PA
CBHW061207070526
44583CB00025B/3148